"Having run inpatient and outpatient eating disorder groups for over 45 years, I expected to have several things to contribute to Carolyn Karoll and Adina Silverman's book *Eating Disorder Group Therapy: A Collaborative Approach*. Reading this book is like taking a superb college course on the topic with a gifted, interesting, and understanding professor. From how to screen applicants, organize a group, facilitate process and content, and deal with innumerable possible problems, these two authors cover everything. They even give the clinician numerous topics to use and how best to present them (materials included)! The detail in this monumental book is fantastic and should prepare a good clinician on best practices for eating disorder group therapy. They even make it look easy. If you ever want to run an eating disorder group, this book is a must. I regularly consult for eating disorder clinicians and treatment programs, and this will be on my recommended reading list."

**Carolyn Costin, MA, MEd, LMFT, CEDS, FAED**, founder of The Carolyn Costin Institute, author of *The Eating Disorder Sourcebook, 8 Keys to Recovery from an Eating Disorder* and more

"What a treasure trove! This book offers the practical strategies and inspiring guidance you need to lead with confidence! If you're looking to amplify the power of group therapy for folks in eating disorder recovery, consider this manual your trusty GPS."

**Rebecca Scritchfield, RDN**, Co-Founder of Self-Care for Diabetes virtual support group and Author of *Body Kindness*

"Eating disorders are healed through connection with others and eating disorder professionals know how challenging it can be to create treatment groups that are successful. Karoll and Silverman have created a step-by-step guidebook that lays out all that a clinician needs to know to create successful and meaningful eating disorder groups to facilitate and foster that essential connection."

**Anna M. Lutz, MPH, RD, CEDS-C**, Lutz, Alexander & Assoc. Nutrition Therapy

"This book strikes a rare balance between offering the 'nuts and bolts' of group work as well as appreciating the soulfulness and meaning of the enterprise. This book is chock full of exercises that any therapist can use to further their work. I find that these exercises enhance group work and help the group to be a meaningful vessel for the deep and meaningful work that each individual in the group must undergo in order to find healing. The book appreciates the depth and nuance of group work without losing sight of the realities and practicalities that make this work possible. In particular, this book is an excellent resource for any therapist who is considering group work as a part of their eating disorders treatment. No eating disorders therapist's shelf is complete without this book."

**Dr. Dana Harron, Psy.D,** Founder, Monarch Wellness & Psychotherapy and author of *Loving Someone with an Eating Disorder*

# Eating Disorder Group Therapy

This is the only book that teaches clinicians how to run an effective, evidence-informed, and multi-disciplinary eating disorder group, incorporating psychoeducation, process group dynamics, and experiential elements.

Whereas group therapy for eating disorders is widely used across many levels of care, the outpatient setting is uniquely poised to deliver effective, multi-disciplinary group therapy. The first part of this book offers practical guidance for conceiving, organizing, and initiating outpatient groups, equipping clinicians with the necessary tools to foster supportive and transformative environments. The second includes seven chapters that delve into the core themes of eating disorder recovery, featuring 60 activities and discussions empowering participants toward growth and resilience. This book teaches clinicians how to collaboratively lead groups to optimize cohesion and harness the collective strength of the group to facilitate change. It provides thorough rationale and psychoeducation for each group exercise and is complete with sample forms, worksheets, and handouts.

Suitable for clinicians and students alike in the eating disorder field, this guide on how to successfully begin and run your own group is a necessary resource.

**Carolyn Karoll, LCSW-C, CEDS-S,** holds a master's in Social Work from the University of Maryland at Baltimore. She has her own private practice in Baltimore, Maryland and is an iaedp™ certified eating disorder specialist and supervisor.

**Adina Silverman, MS, RD, LDN**, holds a master's in Nutrition and Wellness from Benedictine University. She is in private practice in Baltimore, Maryland and specializes in the treatment of eating disorders.

# Eating Disorder Group Therapy

A Collaborative Approach

Carolyn Karoll and Adina Silverman

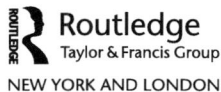
Routledge
Taylor & Francis Group

NEW YORK AND LONDON

Designed cover image: © Getty

First published 2024
by Routledge
605 Third Avenue, New York, NY 10158

and by Routledge
4 Park Square, Milton Park, Abingdon, Oxon, OX14 4RN

*Routledge is an imprint of the Taylor & Francis Group, an informa business.*

*Library of Congress Cataloging-in-Publication Data*
A catalog record for this title has been requested.

ISBN: 978-1-032-55497-6 (hbk)
ISBN: 978-1-032-55495-2 (pbk)
ISBN: 978-1-003-43096-4 (ebk)

DOI: 10.4324/9781003430964

Typeset in Times new Roman
by Apex CoVantage, LLC

To the women of Thrive, past and present, your strength, resilience, and unwavering spirit inspire us daily. This book is dedicated to each of you, for your courage on the path of recovery, your vulnerability in sharing your stories, and your steadfast support for one another. – *CK & AS*

To my beloved mother, Barbara, you were my guiding light, instilling in me the belief that my voice mattered, and empowering me to make a difference. Your love and inspiration are woven into the pages of this book, a testament to your enduring legacy. – *CK*

To my beloved husband and three children, your endless curiosity, laughter, and zest for life remind me to be the best I can be. To push myself to do hard things. To grow. I am blessed to share such a beautiful life with each of you. – *AS*

# Contents

# Notes About the Authors

Carolyn Karoll, LCSW-C, CEDS-S, is a highly regarded therapist with a wealth of qualifications in her field. She holds the distinction of being a Maryland State Board-Certified Licensed Clinical Social Worker, a Maryland State Board of Social Work approved supervisor, a Certified Eating Disorder Specialist, and an Approved Supervisor from the International Association of Eating Disorders Professionals Foundation. She holds a bachelor's degree in Women's Studies (now Gender Studies) from Towson State University, complemented by a master's in Social Work, specializing in clinical mental health from the University of Maryland at Baltimore. She is a member of the National Association of Social Workers and the Academy for Eating Disorders.

Carolyn's extensive experience in the field of eating disorders includes her roles as a family and group therapist at The Center for Eating Disorders at Sheppard Pratt Health System and as the Clinical Supervisor at The Renfrew Center of Baltimore prior to opening her private practice in Towson, Maryland, with a specialized focus on the treatment of eating disorders. Her therapeutic expertise encompasses a broad spectrum, including individual, family, couples, and group therapy. She has leveraged her expertise to present crucial topics such as eating disorder prevention, diagnosis, treatment, group therapy, and body image concerns to mental health professionals as well as the broader community. Her insights have also been featured in print media.

Distinguished by her empathetic approach, Carolyn not only supports her clients, but also educates them about the multifaceted influences that shape their body image and self-esteem. Her commitment extends to helping individuals delve beneath their struggles with food and weight, empowering them to cultivate new mindsets and skills that lead to self-efficacy, self-compassion, and self-acceptance.

Since 2015, Carolyn has co-facilitated the "Thrive" eating disorder recovery group alongside her co-facilitator and co-author, Adina Silverman, MS, RD, LDN. This group serves as a vital support system for women in recovery from eating disorders, guiding them toward achieving harmony in their relationship with food and their bodies. Carolyn's dedication to her profession and her unwavering commitment to the well-being of her clients make her a respected expert in the field of therapy, particularly in the treatment of eating disorders.

Carolyn resides in Baltimore, Maryland with her husband and two boxers.

Carolyn Karoll

Adina Silverman, MS, RD, LDN is a renowned Registered Dietitian specializing in the treatment of eating disorders. She holds a bachelor's degree in Nutritional Sciences from the University of Wisconsin-Madison and a master's in Nutrition and Wellness from Benedictine University. She is a member of the Academy of Nutrition and Dietetics and the Academy for Eating Disorders.

After working in various levels of care in eating disorder treatment programs, Adina began her private practice in Baltimore, Maryland and continues to see clients there. She is passionate about helping adolescents, teenagers, and adults heal their relationships with food and their bodies. She supports her clients to have the courage to cultivate the relationship with food that feels best to them and reject mainstream diet culture messaging. Her thorough and compassionate approach has impacted many individuals and families and distinguished her as a leader in her professional community.

Adina regularly speaks to students, teachers, mental health professionals, and the public on the topics of eating disorders and cultivating healthy relationships with food. She has spoken at professional conferences and been featured in print media and live news broadcasts.

Adina co-facilitates the "Thrive" eating disorder recovery group with her co-author, Carolyn Karoll, LCSW-C, CEDS-S. She is energized by the strength and resilience of the women in this group and firmly believes in the transformative power of group work in eating disorder recovery.

Adina resides in Baltimore, Maryland with her husband and three children.

Adina Silverman

# Preface

We have been leading an outpatient eating disorder group together since 2016. Initially, we did not think long and hard about the decision to co-facilitate our group. We had worked together in a treatment setting for years, worked smoothly together, and had complementary strengths both clinically and professionally. Not long after our group took off, we realized that what began as a way to split the load turned out to benefit our group members profoundly. We provided a more holistic group experience by having the therapist and dietitian in the room at the same time. We each responded to topics brought up or different group members' comments through a different lens. We had additional insights and wisdom to offer to the community. Our group members raved that they had never experienced a group like ours.

We wondered, *Was our group really that much of an outlier?* We knew that creating and running an outpatient eating disorder group took careful consideration, ample planning, and skilled leadership. One cannot simply throw a group together and rush the end result. After realizing that some clinicians were unaware of this or lacked the resources to acquire this knowledge, we decided to disseminate our approach and materials to others.

Mental health clinicians may receive training in facilitating groups, but that training is likely not specific to eating disorder group therapy. Registered Dietitians, on the other hand, may never receive formal support group training. With the rapid growth of private practices in both of our disciplines, it would not be surprising to see an increase in outpatient groups offered. Yet facilitators need an evidence-informed, outcome-driven resource for providing this needed service. We set out on a mission to offer new ideas, creative prompts, and inventive discussions that utilize both clinicians' skill sets and experience. The fruit of that labor is this book.

Eating disorders are isolating illnesses. They sometimes keep sufferers from spending time with loved ones, trying new experiences, or engaging in life in the ways they want to. The precious time of their lives may be tied up looking up calories, compulsively exercising, or hiding away to engage in symptom use. Feelings of disappointment in oneself, or an even stronger sense of shame, form an emotional bunker that is difficult to penetrate. This can feel confining and limiting for some who have been in individual therapy for years. This is why coming together as a group, validating shared struggles, and lifting sufferers out of their isolation has such a profound impact.

Eating disorders are insidious conditions with devastating consequences. It is a harsh reality that eating disorders have the second-highest mortality rates among all mental illnesses, surpassed only by opioid use disorder.[1] The toll is alarming, as one person succumbs to the direct effects of their eating disorder every fifty-two minutes, whether through medical complications or the tragic outcome of suicide.[2]

In the face of this staggering reality, as clinicians, therapists, and Registered Dietitians, we have devoted our lives to helping individuals with eating disorders find their path to recovery. We have witnessed firsthand the profound impact of effective group support on individuals and their families. With great pride and dedication, we present this book as a comprehensive guide for clinicians seeking to establish and lead their own evidence-informed, multidisciplinary eating disorder therapy groups.

A group focusing on specific symptoms alone would naturally alienate some members. This was another reason we felt compelled to write this book. After working in higher levels of care, attending conferences, and reading books pertinent to the field, we wanted to create group exercises that do not assume participants hate food and are restricting food intake or are only in "thin bodies." You will find that the discussions and activities in this book can be used for more than one type of eating disorder, for individuals in larger and smaller bodies, and for all gender identities.

Fast-forward eight years from our first co-facilitated group in 2016. The night of the week has changed, the community members have changed, and even the location has changed to a virtual group (thank you, COVID-19), but the group continues to go strong. The dedicated women who have participated in our group have inspired us, taught us, and pushed us to create group discussions and activities that are meaningful, transformational, and memorable. These women are the inspiration behind this book.

Drawing upon our collective experience of twenty-five years working with individuals struggling with eating disorders and their families, we have led a combined number of eating disorder groups in the thousands. Our passion for supporting those on the path to recovery has fueled our commitment to compile this invaluable resource.

We extend our heartfelt gratitude to the individuals and families who have entrusted us with their journeys toward recovery. We invite readers to join us in using this book's knowledge, experiences, and exercises to guide their outpatient eating disorder groups. Together, we can make a difference in the lives of individuals struggling with eating disorders as we foster connection, empowerment, and healing.

## Notes

1 Arcelus, Jon, Alex J. Mitchell, Jackie Wales, and Søren Nielsen. 2011. "Mortality Rates in Patients with Anorexia Nervosa and Other Eating Disorders." *Archives of General Psychiatry* 68 (7): 724. https://doi.org/10.1001/archgenpsychiatry.2011.74.
2 "Report: Economic Costs of Eating Disorders." *STRIPED*, September 27, 2021. www. hsph.harvard.edu/striped/report-economic-costs-of-eating-disorders/.

# Introduction

Part One of *Eating Disorder Group Therapy: A Collaborative Approach* serves as a manual for the conception, organization, and implementation of successful virtual or in-person outpatient eating disorder groups. It provides clinicians with the tools and strategies to establish and maintain a supportive and transformative group environment. Part Two consists of seven comprehensive chapters covering critical themes in eating disorder recovery. Accompanying activities and discussions empower group participants to explore and address these themes, fostering personal growth and resilience.

Readers of this book will find a subtle focus on the female experience more than other gender identities. However, the activities and discussions are written to allow participation by all gender identities. We focus more on women because the social constructs of gender impose stricter expectations for people identifying as women to conform to these depictions.[1,2]

We hope readers will keep in mind several things as they use this book. For simplicity, the mental health professional will be referred to as "the therapist" and the Registered Dietitian will be referred to as "the dietitian." In the United States, Registered Dietitians go through undergraduate education and beginning in 2024, a graduate degree minimum requirement will be implemented. Registered Dietitians must complete a comprehensive dietetic internship and pass an exam through the Commission on Dietetic Registration to earn this title. While the term "nutritionist" is often used to refer to a Registered Dietitian and is a legally regulated term in most states, it can sometimes refer to someone who has very little, if any, higher education in the field of dietetics. Professionals working with individuals with eating disorders should always encourage their patients to work with a Registered Dietitian.

The use of "therapist" throughout this book refers to a mental health professional specializing in diagnosing and treating eating disorders. This typically requires a master's degree in clinical social work, psychology, marriage and family therapy, counseling or a doctorate in psychology followed by requirements of their licensing board.

DOI: 10.4324/9781003430964-1

We use the phrase "larger bodies" in reference to a body type. We are aware of the potentially problematic nature of this term, as it implies "larger than" something. We use this term as a neutral descriptor and an adjective, not a judgment. In her groundbreaking book *Fat Talk: Parenting in the Age of Diet Culture*, journalist Virginia Sole-Smith endorses that individuals in larger bodies should choose and use the descriptor they identify with instead of others choosing these labels for them.[3] Following suit, we recommend that group facilitators ask about and honor the language that resonates with the group members, whether that be fat, larger-bodied, or plus-sized, just to name a few.

Throughout the book, we make a distinction between discussions and activities. Discussions are solely conversation-based; they do not require using materials or having members complete worksheets, make lists, or engaging in any other experiential task. Conversely, activities involve something more than discussion. This varies from completing a worksheet to engaging in a body scan. We hope this distinction allows group facilitators to effectively distinguish between the different exercises and easily select what they are looking for.

There is a gray box with a prompt or question inside for most activities and discussions. This feature is meant to allow group facilitators or other readers of this book to quickly identify the prompt or "gist" of a specific discussion or activity without having to read the full instructions. While other questions are posed later in the discussion or activity to further the group's conversation, the material in the gray box is intended to capture the focus of that particular exercise for quick reference.

With each discussion or activity, several discussion questions are meant to help group facilitators commence, guide, and deepen the conversation. We pose many questions throughout this book that can be used in group discussions, but we hope that group facilitators will use this less as a script and more as a roadmap in each exercise. One of the joys of leading our groups is seeing the organic twists and turns that discussions take. We provide group facilitators with enough background information and structure to begin each exercise. We do not provide answers or expected answers to each discussion question, as the answers will vary from group to group.

For activities, all materials needed to run the activity are listed. Clarification is provided when materials differ depending on whether the group is in-person or virtual. Virtual group facilitators are encouraged to familiarize themselves with features available through virtual conferencing platforms, such as screen share and group chat, which are necessary to lead many of the activities in this book without any physical materials.

Readers will find a special section called the Facilitators' Forum at the end of each discussion or activity in this book. This dedicated section is designed to provide support and enhance the facilitation process. Within this section, readers will discover valuable tips, recommendations, and practical strategies to create a dynamic and impactful group environment. Drawing from our own experiences and insights, we offer guidance on navigating challenges, fostering meaningful engagement, and cultivating a supportive atmosphere for participants.

## Notes

1 Piran, Niva. 2017. *Journeys of Embodiment at the Intersection of Body and Culture the Developmental Theory of Embodiment.* Saint Louis: Elsevier Science.
2 Wolf, Naomi. 1991. *The Beauty Myth: How Images of Beauty are Used Against Women.* New York: W. Morrow.
3 Sole-Smith, Virginia. 2023. *Fat Talk: Parenting in the Age of Diet Culture.* New York: Henry Holt and Company.

# Part I

# Chapter 1

# The Role of the Multidisciplinary-Led Group in Outpatient Treatment for Eating Disorders

## A Comprehensive Overview

> I have felt "normal" and understood at the end of each group and have also found myself doing some soul-searching as a result of conversation or questions asked by group members. I have been inspired, motivated, encouraged, and, most importantly, challenged by each member in different ways. This group and the women in it have shown me in their own special ways how to begin to love myself and heal.
>
> — Former group member

Eating disorders thrive in isolation, making a supportive community vital for recovery. Group therapy offers a powerful approach, enabling individuals to connect, share experiences, and support one another on their path to healing. This chapter provides a comprehensive guide to understanding the pivotal role of group therapy in treating eating disorders in the outpatient setting.

This chapter explores the distinctive features of outpatient groups, highlighting their differences from higher levels of care. Considerations for in-person and virtual group formats and practical strategies are offered to facilitators to create inclusive and welcoming environments that foster engagement and trust. The benefits of a multidisciplinary approach are emphasized, showcasing the collaborative partnership between therapists and Registered Dietitians as an innovative and effective means of leading these groups.

Furthermore, this chapter addresses the evolving landscape of virtual group therapy, which has gained significant prominence following the COVID-19 pandemic. The benefits, challenges, and best practices for implementing virtual group therapy are examined, providing practitioners with insights to navigate this evolving treatment modality effectively.

## Group Therapy in Eating Disorder Recovery: Breaking Isolation

Eating disorders create an inherently isolating experience as they thrive and persist in secrecy, irrespective of their specific symptomology. The pervasive shame

DOI: 10.4324/9781003430964-3

associated with that secrecy and the enduring stigma surrounding eating disorders further compounds the isolation experienced by so many.

Group therapy is an essential component of comprehensive eating disorder treatment. Eating disorder support groups provide a space for members to relate to one another, reducing feelings of isolation and enhancing motivation to recover.[1]

When individuals enter eating disorder treatment, the transformative power of finding a supportive community of people who "get it" becomes evident. By sharing their stories and experiences, group members discover a profound sense of connection, realizing they are not alone in their struggles. Together, they inspire each other to confront the societal pressures and obstacles perpetuated by a culture that idealizes restrictive diets and thin bodies.

A safe and accepting environment is created in group therapy, fostering compassion and validation among members. This nurturing atmosphere promotes the development of skills such as self-compassion and self-validation, which are fundamental in the journey of eating disorder recovery. Additionally, group therapy offers an opportunity for interpersonal growth. Members are encouraged to practice vulnerability within the safety of the group setting, creating an environment where they can provide and receive support and accountability throughout their recovery process.

## Group Thertapy Across Levels of Care

Group therapy is offered in all levels of care, from inpatient treatment centers and residential programs to Partial Hospitalization Programs (PHP), Intensive Outpatient Programs (IOP), and outpatient settings. Despite the prevalence of group therapy in treating eating disorders, there is little guidance on this subject. This book focuses on outpatient groups and is intended to be a resource to support professionals. Its purpose is to provide support and guidance in forming meaningful groups that enrich the therapeutic experience, ultimately fostering healing and growth for individuals receiving outpatient treatment.

Treatment needs differ depending on the acuity of symptoms. Groups for patients conducted in higher levels of care typically focus on developing motivation to change, medical stabilization, and cessation of eating disorder symptoms. Higher levels of care require intense, exhausting work as one may be undergoing meal plan advancement or experiencing physical symptoms, including constipation, edema, and night sweats. For others, blocking urges to binge or exercise stirs up overwhelming emotions that the use of these symptoms has suppressed. Many of these patients are not ready to begin the work of body acceptance or build the skills to live in a diet-centered culture with narrow beauty ideals.

Patients in outpatient groups are typically ready for a more psychodynamic, experiential approach. Once a person receives adequate, consistent nutritional intake and does not regularly engage in their symptoms, such as restricting, bingeing, purging, or excessively exercising, there is space to "dig deeper" into the psychological underpinnings of the disorder. As they begin to experience what it feels like not engaging in these behaviors, a rich landscape of psychological work presents itself. Individual therapy is undoubtedly the primary place where this work occurs. Still, the group therapy setting can further the process by allowing one to explore these topics alongside others going through similar struggles. Hearing group members verbalize thoughts or core beliefs that they have only said aloud within the walls of their therapist or dietitian's office can be validating and shame-reducing.

Combining the wisdom of an eating disorder therapist and a Registered Dietitian reinforces the message that eating disorders are simultaneously about food and weight and not about food and weight. The dietitian can speak to the nutritional and physiological processes of the eating disorder and correct inaccuracies in beliefs or thoughts around metabolism, nutritional needs, and body trust. The therapist has expertise in facilitating discussions around psychological themes in recovery, such as the frequently experienced emotions and beliefs that people may hold about themselves and the world around them. In this unique partnership, the therapist and dietitian can cultivate discussion around meaningful themes in recovery, bringing awareness to emotions, feelings, and core beliefs while connecting these topics to how they perceive their relationship with food and their bodies.

## Group Modalities

There are various types of groups utilized to treat eating disorders. The most common types are psychoeducational groups, process groups, and groups focusing on a specific evidenced-based modality, including but not limited to Cognitive Behavioral Therapy (CBT) and Dialectical Behavior Therapy (DBT). Additionally, there are groups dedicated to providing education and support to families/support persons (with or without the identified patient present) and groups devoted to nutrition education and meal support.

We have discovered that combining psychoeducation, experiential approaches, and evidence-based and evidence-informed modalities offers an innovative and effective way to treat eating disorders. This book provides a comprehensive integration of various therapeutic techniques from CBT, DBT, Acceptance and Commitment Therapy (ACT), Solution-Focused Therapy (SFT), Narrative Therapy, Motivational Interviewing (MI), Positive Psychology, Compassion-Focused Therapy (CFT), Mindfulness-Based Stress Reduction (MBSRN), and other mindfulness-based approaches, along with insights from Attachment Theory. The principles of Health at Every Size® (HAES) and a social justice and feminist framework guide our work and serve as the foundation for our approach.

## In-Person Groups

### Environment

When most people think of in-person support groups, they probably have the image of a group of plastic chairs situated in a circle and a refreshment table sitting off to the side. This image is far from the setting we provided as we ran our in-person outpatient eating disorder group for years before the COVID-19 pandemic. Imagine a warmly lit room with several cozy couches and chairs that were, as you guessed, arranged in a circle. Small touches like an aromatherapy diffuser and hand lotion were present to make the space feel pleasing and welcoming. The simple act of applying hand lotion may seem trivial, but inviting our group members to slow down and mindfully inhabit their bodies for the duration of the group allowed a moment to relax and notice tense shoulders, dry hands, or hungry bellies.

After a few years, we began offering snacks in the middle of our circle to help group members practice eating in front of one another and work through the shame or embarrassment that some felt when doing this. Our group ran close to dinner time, so providing snacks normalized some group members' hunger during this hour.

Group facilitators should consider their group members when providing snacks during the group. Does anyone have an allergy? Are there nutrition labels on the food or nutrition claims on the packaging that may be triggering to members? Does anyone require kosher or halal-certified foods? Part of creating a safe and nurturing environment is providing food that everyone has the opportunity to eat. Taking food out of the packaging and putting it in decorative containers can reduce the fixation on grams of carbs, sugar, fat, or calories, helping to reduce guilt or shame.

When providing in-person groups, consider seating options. Individuals who struggle with eating disorders come in all shapes and sizes. Less than six percent of people diagnosed with eating disorders are regarded as medically "underweight."[2] Providing seating that can accommodate a wide range of body shapes and sizes and a variety of seating options is preferable to providing one kind of seat. Making seating comfortable and secure requires considering weight limits, accessibility, and dimensions. It was not uncommon for our group members to shuffle themselves around before the start of the group so that everyone could sit where they were most comfortable. Interestingly, we noticed that this became one of the rituals that helped the group feel connected as people started leaving certain seats open for group members in their preferred spots.

We also encourage inviting members to provide feedback about the group environment. We often asked whether members preferred overhead lighting or soft lights supplied with lamps, electric candles, and accent lighting around the room. It is important to be mindful of individual sensitivities and potential triggers, such as traumatic memories or allergies, which may inform the decision to incorporate certain scents in the group setting.

### Bodies in the Room

There is great value in having an in-person group, specifically an eating disorder group, as so much discussion encompasses thoughts and fears around one's body. Seeing someone's body as they describe their experience in their skin provides a layer of intimacy and a deeper understanding of how someone sees themself. Sharing the room, and quite literally the space their bodies hold, allows for a closeness that can be hard to cultivate when group members are behind a screen and only seen from their shoulders up.

When discussing one's body in the presence of others, the discomfort of opening up and being vulnerable can intensify. Being physically present allows group members to explore their beliefs and attitudes toward individuals with diverse bodies and challenge any weight- or size-based or other prejudiced assumptions they may hold. The aim is to foster an environment where group members are seen and valued beyond their physical appearance.

## Virtual Groups

### Evolution of the Virtual Format

The United States faced the beginning of the COVID-19 pandemic in March 2020, causing how we worked, socialized, and interacted with one another to take a different form. At the same time as work shifted online and socialization occurred through screens, the emergence of virtual treatment and support evolved rather quickly. Treatment programs offered virtual programming options within months of the pandemic's onset. Outpatient providers were holding telehealth sessions. Support groups that were meeting in person began to meet virtually.

The precautions required to mitigate the spread of COVID-19 in many ways created an environment ripe for developing eating disorders. Pandemic-induced isolation, increased media consumption, and damaging "wellness" messaging profoundly impacted individuals, especially those struggling with eating disorders.

A 2022 study identified various risk factors for individuals with eating disorders, which significantly escalated during the pandemic. Among these factors was a notable surge in media and social media consumption, particularly concerning the dissemination of fatphobic messaging. Additionally, limited access to healthcare services, altered food availability, and restrictions on physical exercise further contributed to the heightened risk experienced by individuals with eating disorders.[3] During the pandemic, the fear of weight gain (the "Quarantine 15") and other fatphobic messaging were even more rampant, posing a significant risk to those already struggling with an eating disorder.

In the absence of being able to sit in a meeting or support group with others, the use of virtual platforms for connecting boomed. Support groups were no different, and those with eating disorders needed urgent support. After realizing that our worlds as we knew them would not return to normal in a couple of weeks or months, we changed our in-person group to a virtual platform. In our experience, this shift was well-accepted by our group members as meeting through screens had become the norm.

### Environment

Creating an optimal virtual group environment can be challenging due to participants joining from different locations. However, group facilitators can still influence certain factors to enhance the group experience. Facilitators should review the following guidelines with incoming participants and ensure that they are clearly communicated to virtual group members before their first group session.

Ask participants to join the virtual group from a location with a reliable and strong internet connection. While it is not always within their control, a stable connection minimizes disruptions such as poor audio quality, delays, or technical difficulties that can detract from the sensitive and confidential nature of the discussions.

It is crucial to ensure that participants have privacy for the duration of the virtual group. While one of the advantages of a virtual group is the ability for members to join from various locations, such as a hotel room in Hawaii or a study room in a campus library, it is essential to emphasize that they should never join from a setting where their privacy is compromised or where others can be heard or seen in the background.

Joining a virtual group from a public or non-private location can lead to distractions and violate the group's confidentiality. Such distractions can diminish the sense of safety and comfort for other members. Therefore, it is important to communicate the importance of selecting a private environment where individuals can freely express themselves without concerns about being overheard or observed.

Some groups ask that members not mute themselves or turn off their cameras while they are not talking. Keeping themselves unmuted facilitates the sense that the group is sitting together. Just like one cannot mute themself or keep others from seeing them while sitting in a room, they should not be able to when in a virtual room with the group. This request also helps ensure that members are not listening to anything in the background or engaging in something that would take their attention away from the group.

While we have identified some advantages to having actual "bodies in the room," some members find that the limited view from a screen reduces the intensity of their urges to compare their bodies to those of their peers. This limited view gives them the experience of feeling seen for who they are and less worried that judgments about their body size or shape will influence their interactions.

It is common for those struggling with eating disorders and associated comorbidities to see themselves from a spectator's point of view. Depending on the Health Insurance Portability and Accountability Act (HIPAA)-compliant platform you are using, members may be able to hide their view of themselves on the screen while still allowing others to see them, which may prevent self-objectification. Self-objectification is a process that occurs when women think about and treat themselves as objects to be regarded and evaluated based on appearance; it is a risk factor for the development of eating disorders.[4] For group members who struggle with self-objectification, we suggest concealing one's self-view to foster a more embodied experience.

## The Dietitian and Therapist Partnership

Benefits of having a dietitian and therapist co-facilitate a group, beyond merging their knowledge bases, include modeling interpersonal relationships and mitigating "burn-out" or compassion fatigue. Co-facilitation fosters a more dynamic engagement, allowing a facilitator to take the lead in supporting the discussion. Co-facilitation permits the other to be more attuned to group dynamics, such as members' responses and needs. An example of this could include a member's body language suddenly changing from attentive and engaged to avoiding eye contact and slumped posture, which one facilitator may be more attuned to than the other leading the discussion.

While support groups are not always professionally moderated, multidisciplinary facilitation is an asset to group members. Online support groups that professional facilitators did not lead were found to be effective in a 2009 study.[5] However, the positive role of a professional facilitator in promoting trust and a sense of safety in the group and providing vital psycho-educational information and support to the participants has also been found.[6] Our experience co-leading a group for almost a decade supports these findings. The therapist and dietitian partnership provides the optimal opportunity to address underlying issues and the members' relationship with food and their body, the two primary aspects of the eating disorder.[7]

While the therapist and dietitian will be expected to further discussions by asking open-ended questions, summarizing and clarifying information, and providing validation and empathy, they will also be tasked with introducing topics and making connections related to their area of expertise. For instance, a dietitian may take the lead in discussing nutrition myths. The therapist's role would include helping members tap into the function of holding onto a dietary rule even when there is evidence to debunk it. In another example, if the group addresses interpersonal relationships, the therapist may begin by asking members to identify traits that make a relationship healthy versus unhealthy. The dietitian could ask members to notice how their criteria for healthy and unhealthy relationships with people are similar to how they speak of their relationship with food and their bodies.

In a 2020 study, participants of professionally led support groups reported that facilitators who were both assertive and compassionate instilled trust and a sense of safety in the group.[8] The assertiveness in moderating and steering the conversation in the right direction while managing triggering language made them feel safe to share their experiences in the group. Most participants appreciated feeling emotionally supported by the facilitators' compassionate, non-judgmental stance.

Given the stigma and shame people with eating disorders often experience, they may hesitate to trust others. It follows that to ensure trust, safety, and retention in group participation, facilitators must have knowledge of and training on eating disorders, regardless of their discipline.

Much overlap exists regarding therapists' and dietitians' roles in eating disorder group facilitation. Both require understanding eating disorders and knowledge of group processes, dynamics, and facilitation. We strongly recommend potential group facilitators develop that knowledge and skill set before starting a group.

## Notes

1  Waller, Archana, Chiara Paganini, Katrina Andrews, and Vicki Hutton. 2020. "The Experience of Adults Recovering from an Eating Disorder in Professionally-Led Support Groups." *Qualitative Research Journal* 21 (2): 217–229. https://doi.org/10.1108/qrj-07-2020-0088.
2  "Eating Disorder Statistics: General & Diversity Stats." *National Association of Anorexia Nervosa and Associated Disorders.* https://anad.org/eating-disorders-statistics/.
3  Cooper, Marita, Erin E. Reilly, Jaclyn A. Siegel, Kathryn Coniglio, Shiri Sadeh-Sharvit, Emily M. Pisetsky, and Lisa M. Anderson. 2022. "Eating Disorders during the COVID-19 Pandemic and Quarantine: An Overview of Risks and Recommendations for Treatment and Early Intervention." *Eating Disorders* 30 (1): 54–76. https://doi.org/10.1080/10640266.2020.1790271.
4  Fredrickson, Barbara L., and Tomi-Ann Roberts. 1997. "Objectification Theory: Toward Understanding Women's Lived Experiences and Mental Health Risks." *Psychology of Women Quarterly* 21 (2): 173–206. https://doi.org/10.1111/j.1471-6402.1997.tb00108.x.
5  McCormack, Abby, and Neil S. Coulson. 2009. "Individuals with Eating Disorders and the Use of Online Support Groups as a Form of Social Support." *Cyberpsychology: Journal of Psychosocial Research on Cyberspace* 3 (2): Article 5. https://cyberpsychology.eu/article/view/4228.

6 Lefley, Harriet P. 2009. "A Psychoeducational Support Group for Serious Mental Illness." *The Journal for Specialists in Group Work* 34 (4): 369–81. https://doi.org/10.1080/01933920903219094.

7 Mitchell, Sharon L., Jessalyn Klein, and Althea Maduramente. 2014. "Assessing the Impact of an Eating Disorders Treatment Team Approach with College Students." *Eating Disorders* 23 (1): 45–59. https://doi.org/10.1080/10640266.2014.959847.

8 Waller, Paganini, Andrews, and Hutton, "The Experience of Adults."

Chapter 2

# Forming an Outpatient Eating Disorder Group

## Recruitment, Screening, and Practical Considerations

The efficacy of an outpatient eating disorder group is intricately tied to the work done on the front end, encompassing considerations such as recruitment, group composition, format selection, and policy development. This chapter delves into these critical aspects, exploring the factors that lay the groundwork for a successful and impactful group.

With a strong emphasis on inclusivity and fostering cohesion, the screening process takes into account various factors such as age, gender identification, life stages, motivation level, and medical stability. These considerations play a vital role in shaping the group's effectiveness and ensuring that it meets the unique needs of the participants.

The chapter examines the advantages and disadvantages of in-person and virtual group formats, providing insights for making an informed decision on the most suitable approach. It also tackles the determination of the optimal group size and the deliberation between an ongoing or fixed-session format.

Additionally, the chapter addresses the importance of establishing clear group policies to create a safe and supportive environment. By setting guidelines and expectations, these policies contribute to the overall efficacy of the group and foster a sense of trust among participants.

Financial aspects related to billing will also be addressed, offering a practical understanding of the financial considerations involved in the group formation process. Appendices provide valuable resources, including a sample participant application and an Informed Consent document. These resources aim to support the practical implementation of the group formation process.

## Part One: Considerations for Group Composition

### Inclusion and Exclusion Criteria

Although stereotypes around eating disorders frequently associate them with young, white, privileged women, they affect people of all gender identities, ages, socioeconomic statuses, and life stages. Proper inclusion and exclusion criteria

DOI: 10.4324/9781003430964-4

provide specificity to the group community to optimize cohesion. Therefore, group facilitators must clearly understand what their group will offer and the demographics they aim to serve. In the next chapter, we will explain why we do not universally recommend diagnosis-specific groups and caution against using diagnosis as part of the exclusion criteria. The thoughtful screening takes a little more of the group facilitators' time on the front end, but the benefits of cohesion and retention are invaluable outcomes.

### Age

Setting a minimum age limit or age range for the group can help members bond and begin to feel they have something in common. Being sensitive to the ages of those in the group and how broad the age inclusion criteria web is cast is critical for providing developmentally appropriate care. Setting firm and protective age-related exclusion criteria can help shield those who are more impressionable and cultivate a space where members can relate to one another. A woman in her forties in a group of teenagers or college-aged women may feel like an outlier who's not understood by others, which can jeopardize her retention.

### Gender Identification

Although many people imagine an eating disorder support group consisting of cis women only, eating disorders undeniably affect people across the entire gender spectrum. All of these people are deserving of support. The benefit of an all-female group community has been recognized for decades, as many women find it uncomfortable to discuss insecurities about their appearance, including their body shape and size, in front of men.

Eating disorders also affect men and are estimated to comprise 10–20% of cases. However, the prevalence is likely higher due to the well-known underdiagnosis of eating disorders in men.[1] Many people regard eating disorders as a "female problem," which only adds to the shame and stigma men may feel about coming forward with their struggles. To create a safe space for men to seek and receive support, facilitators should consider groups offered only to males if they have expertise in this area.

There are many groups open to all gender identifications that run successfully. However, those who do not identify as male or female, as well as transgender adults and adolescents, often feel marginalized and are subject to greater discrimination.[2] A 2022 study of college-aged students found the risk for developing an eating disorder risk is significantly higher in the genderqueer and nonconforming community.[3] A 2015 study found that transgender college students were more than four times more likely to report an eating disorder diagnosis than their cisgender female counterparts.[4] Given the high prevalence of eating disorders within this community and their marginalized status in the broader population, it is important to prioritize the provision of group therapy tailored specifically to their needs.

### Life Stages

Gearing a group toward middle schoolers differs greatly from designing one for college students or individuals in mid-life or late life. Understanding the target demographic will guide everything from the activities selection to the group meeting time.

We recommend separating adolescents and younger teenagers from adults in outpatient eating disorder groups to tailor interventions to better meet the specific needs of each life stage. Adolescents and younger teenagers are often most comfortable opening up to peers and may feel inhibited in a group of adults. Adolescents are highly susceptible to peer influence. Therapy can leverage positive peer influence to encourage healthier behaviors and attitudes by placing them in a group with other adolescents. Seeing their peers progress, share coping strategies, and engage in recovery-oriented activities can inspire adolescents to actively participate in their own recovery.

There is a common misconception that eating disorders are illnesses that impact only teenagers and young adults. Consequently, mid- or late-life individuals may feel ashamed and discouraged from seeking treatment. If they seek treatment – in this case, group therapy – they often think they cannot relate to the younger group members. Creating a support group tailored to these life stages could help alleviate the shame they feel and increase the likelihood of them seeking and receiving appropriate treatment. Such groups can address the unique bio-psycho-social and relational aspects of eating disorders in later life.[5]

### Stage of Recovery

Outpatient groups are typically designed for individuals needing ongoing support to maintain their recovery. Regardless of their stage in this process, it is vital for prospective group members to recognize and acknowledge their eating disorders as a problem and to exhibit a strong motivation to bring about meaningful change. A willingness to participate in the group process, a desire to learn and practice new skills, and a commitment to working toward recovery are all critical factors in determining whether someone is an appropriate candidate for an outpatient eating disorder group.

Not all individuals with eating disorders are suitable candidates for outpatient group therapy. A higher level of care, such as an inpatient program, residential treatment, or partial hospitalization, may be necessary for applicants who are medically unstable, require intensive monitoring or support, or pose a risk of harm to themselves or others. If a higher level of care is recommended, the individual will undergo a comprehensive assessment by a qualified healthcare provider to determine the most suitable level of care for their specific needs and provide them with the necessary support and treatment.

### Group Setting

Virtual treatment options became increasingly common during the COVID-19 pandemic and continue to be accepted by clinicians and individuals seeking treatment. Virtual treatment allows facilitators to collaborate despite physical distance. On the other hand, many individuals seek in-person support after interacting virtually for so long. Facilitators can choose between in-person and virtual group options when forming a group; there is value in both options.

In the second part of this book, we present adaptations for group discussions and activities which may be implemented for both in-person and virtual group settings.

### Group Size

While different sources and experts may provide varying recommendations based on their clinical experience and theoretical perspectives, there is no definitive consensus regarding the optimal group therapy size. In most cases, research suggests that groups should ideally consist of no more than ten participants.[6] Factors such as the therapeutic approach, specific goals of the group, the demands on the facilitators, and the population being treated can influence opinions on group size. The minimum group size is determined by the necessary number of individuals for cohesive functioning, while the maximum group size is determined by the therapist's capacity to work effectively with participants within the allotted time frame.[7] However, it is important to note that large group sizes may negatively affect attendance rate if group members begin to feel that the group is so large their absence will go unnoticed.

Group size should strike a balance between creating a safe and supportive environment for individual engagement and fostering a sense of community and diverse perspectives. As mentioned earlier, optimal group size may vary based on practical aspects such as physical space and available resources. It may require ongoing assessment and adjustment based on feedback and the evolving needs of the group members.

### Ongoing or Fixed-Session Format

When deciding between an ongoing or fixed-session format, facilitators should consider various factors such as treatment goals, the patient's needs, and available resources. It is important to note that the effectiveness of both formats can be influenced by other factors, such as group size, facilitator expertise, participant engagement, and the integration of evidence-based treatment approaches.

Consider the needs and preferences of the individuals participating in the group. Some participants may benefit from continued support and the sense of community that comes with an ongoing format. Facilitators must consider the group's evolving needs in an ongoing group and tailor their interventions accordingly.

In contrast, others may prefer a structured program with a fixed duration and specific focus. These types of groups are often designed to target particular skills or topics (i.e., DBT for binge eating or intuitive eating), making them more appealing to individuals who have a specific area of interest or want to address certain challenges. A fixed-session group is also advantageous when offered at opportune times for certain populations: for example, a six-week support group for college students over winter break.

With either group structure, the availability of the facilitators will influence what type of group is offered. An ongoing format requires ongoing availability and commitment from facilitators, while a fixed-session format may be more manageable in terms of scheduling.

Considering the flexibility and adaptability of the group as it pertains to members entering and leaving will also impact the type of group facilitators choose. An ongoing format allows new members to join and others to leave as needed, offering a continuous support system. A fixed-session format provides a clear start and end point, allowing participants to plan accordingly and ensuring a sense of closure.

Additionally, the affordability of the group is an important consideration. In general, fixed-session formats may be more cost-effective as they have a predetermined duration. Participants can plan and budget accordingly, knowing the total cost of the group upfront. This can be advantageous for individuals with limited financial resources. Ongoing formats involve regular sessions over an extended period, accumulating higher costs over time. However, the affordability of an ongoing format can also depend on factors such as the frequency of sessions, the payment structure (i.e., weekly or monthly), and any potential discounts or financial assistance available.

## Recruiting New Members

Member recruitment involves advertising the group, communicating with potential members, and distributing an application to screen members. There are countless places to get the word out about a group actively recruiting new members. However, facilitators should think about their target group population and tailor their efforts accordingly.

Utilizing professional listservs or social media groups allows facilitators to reach a broad audience and expand outreach effectively. In doing so, they can familiarize themselves with other clinicians and widen their referral network. Refer to Appendix 2A for a sample clinician referral form.

An application should be sent once a potential group member reaches out to the facilitators. Refer to Appendix 2B for a sample application. Although written for an adult female group, it can be easily modified for a different target demographic. Provide clear instructions for the applicant to return the form. Facilitators should review the application and discuss whether or not to proceed with screening the potential member.

## Screening New Members

As facilitators start recruiting new group members, they must understand how to evaluate the applications and conduct screening to ensure the appropriate selection of individuals for the group. This evaluation and screening phase is integral to the group formation process and will vary depending on the specific type of group being formed. Both facilitators should review the application. We recommend contacting an applicant even if they are not an appropriate fit for the group. Doing so allows them to know that their application was received and to continue looking for a group that is a more appropriate fit.

For most outpatient eating disorder support groups, facilitators will want to ensure applicants have an outpatient team, that their symptom use does not warrant a higher level of care, and that their expectations for the group are aligned with what is offered. The screening criteria may vary slightly for a group that caters to a different demographic.

If an applicant looks like a good fit for the group, they move to the next phase of screening. Facilitators have a choice in how to proceed. One option is to require a screening phone call, about fifteen minutes on average, with that applicant. This phone call allows the group facilitators to get to know this individual better, hear more about where they are in their recovery process, and field the applicant's questions about the group. Sample questions that group facilitators may ask during a screening call are listed in Figure 2.1.

Facilitators may also choose to do a full assessment with the applicant. A complete assessment is a more thorough way to get to know the applicant and is preferred by some clinicians. The therapist or the dietitian could conduct this assessment. It must be communicated to the applicant that this appointment is billed the same way as an intake appointment. Facilitators should be mindful that this option may be cost-prohibitive for many people.

Whether facilitators choose a phone call or assessment, this step is a type of "pre-group preparation."[8] This is fundamental in optimizing group efficacy, cohesion, and focus. When group members feel prepared and have the opportunity to understand what to expect from the group, they are likely to "show an increased amount of faith in the group as a whole."[9]

**Sample Questions for Screening Calls**

- How would you describe where you are in your recovery process?
- Have you ever participated in group therapy before?
- How long have you been struggling with disordered eating or a diagnosed eating disorder?
- How frequently are you engaging in eating disorder symptoms? (To assess the acuity of eating disorder symptoms, probing questions about symptom use are appropriate).
- Have you received any treatment for your eating disorder? If so, what kind and for how long?
- What motivated you to seek support from an eating disorder support group at this time?
- Are you currently under the care of healthcare or mental health professionals for your eating disorder? If so, who comprises your team?
- What are your expectations and goals for participating in the group?
- Are you willing to commit to attending the group for at least [minimum number of] weeks?

*Figure 2.1* Sample questions to ask during a screening phone call with a prospective group member.

Screening calls are a time to invite prospective group members to ask questions about the group. They may have questions about the group's size, makeup, or structure. Answering these questions thoroughly and honestly helps the individual set accurate expectations for what to expect in their first session. This dialogue also builds trust in the group facilitators, setting the tone for a positive group therapy experience.

We aim for transparency in volunteering certain information during these screening calls as it can help optimize group cohesion, something we will discuss more in Chapter 4. For example, if the group community has an average member age of twenty-five at a particular time and an application is received from a forty-five-year-old, we would tell this to the prospective member during this screening call. Being transparent regarding what the incoming member can expect helps build trust and allows them to consider if they would be comfortable in the community. While we are confident in our ability to lead a group of varied ages, sometimes individuals seeking outpatient support know what type of community they seek. Being honest about the group's makeup helps that individual enter group with realistic expectations or continue searching for a group that better matches their needs.

### Outpatient Team

Outpatient group therapy is not a replacement for higher levels of care, individual therapy, or nutritional counseling; therefore, all group members should have an established outpatient treatment team before starting the group. Having an outpatient team is non-negotiable in our group (for safety and liability purposes); however, depending on the type of group, group facilitators may decide that it is permissible for a group member not to have a full team.

### Billing and Financial Considerations

Although collaborative group therapy benefits our group members, it is still a professional service for which members pay a predetermined fee. Group facilitators should fully understand that co-facilitated groups provide a comprehensive service and price their group accordingly. Remember that there are not one but two clinicians practicing, and the group should be financially beneficial for each professional. Facilitators should consider the length of each group session, rates of competing outpatient groups, and the size of the group to set an appropriate per-person rate for the group.

Clinicians who are out-of-network providers may provide a "superbill" to the participants after each group. The "superbill" is a form that contains an itemized list of services provided to a patient. Depending on the clinicians' policy, the group members would need to submit this form to their insurance company, or the office may submit it on their behalf. If a "superbill" is provided, the group facilitators must ensure that the member understands that a superbill is *not* a guarantee of reimbursement from the insurance company. Members must inquire about their out-of-network benefits and understand their reimbursement rates and conditions.

### Billing Schedules

Billing schedules may differ based on whether a group operates as a closed cohort with a fixed session duration or as a closed, rolling admission group. For the former, we recommend collecting payment in full by the start of the first group. Collecting payment upfront has several advantages. First, it ensures everyone is paid in full, negating the need for any further bookkeeping. Second, not collecting payment during group or checking members' balances preserves group time. Lastly, when a group member pays in full for a fixed number of group sessions, they may feel more invested in the entire group experience. In Chapter 4, we will discuss some group members' fears of entering a group community and the challenge of building a cohesive group where everyone feels they belong. If someone pays per group and does not feel that the group is the right fit for them, they may be more inclined to drop out at the first sign of discomfort. We have found that group members typically need a few sessions to feel comfortable.

An eating disorder can be a very costly illness. If paying for all groups upfront would pose a financial hardship for someone, group facilitators should exercise their discretion in negotiating a feasible payment plan that accommodates both parties. It is important to consider that group members may also have financial obligations for psychiatry, therapy, and nutrition appointments. Being understanding and flexible regarding the group member's financial responsibility is a kindness extended when possible.

Payment may be collected at each session for an ongoing rolling admission group. Facilitators may request an electronic form of payment on file, such as a credit card, and charge each member's card after the group.

### Attendance and Billing

In a fixed-session group, we strongly recommend that all members commit to paying for the entire cycle, irrespective of any planned or unplanned absences. Viewing the group cycle as a package offer helps prevent negotiations over fees in cases of illness, forgetting to attend a group session, or having other commitments that hinder their participation. It is also the fairest method as it does not require making special arrangements "just this one time" or risk other group members feeling slighted if they feel they have not been allowed the same entitlement.

For ongoing groups, it is the responsibility of the group facilitators to determine the method of charging for absences. In our group, we generally waive the group fee if a member provides at least 24-hour notice of their absence or if there is an emergency. The definition of an emergency is at the discretion of the facilitators but should be communicated to potential members before they join the group. It is essential to set this boundary as facilitators dedicate their time during the workday to the group. Like individual therapy or nutrition appointments, running a business where services are provided without compensation is not sustainable.

Additionally, it would be unfair to group members who consistently attend to find themselves in suboptimal group sizes. Whatever billing policy the group facilitators agree upon should be clearly stated in the Informed Consent and Financial Agreement forms. Verbal communication of this policy to new members is also recommended. By establishing clear guidelines for attendance and billing, we create a transparent and equitable framework that supports the group's sustainability while respecting the facilitators' and members' needs and commitments.

### Preparing New Members

Once facilitators agree to accept an applicant into the group as a new member, they should send the Informed Consent and other relevant forms, including a Financial Agreement, Group Rules, and a Release of Information for Outpatient Providers. The Informed Consent is a thorough document that explains essential details about group therapy and advises the group member on appropriate engagement in the group. Please refer to Appendix 2C for a sample Informed Consent written for an adult women's group.

In addition, it is essential for group facilitators to review the Informed Consent and Group Rules with new members. This review ensures that they understand the expectations and guidelines. In the upcoming chapter, Table 3.1 lists standard group rules for an eating disorder support group. Facilitators are encouraged to personalize these rules to align with the specific dynamics of their group.

## Notes

1 Sweeting, Helen, Laura Walker, Alice MacLean, Chris Patterson, Ulla Räisänen, and Kate Hunt. 2015. "Prevalence of Eating Disorders in Males: A Review of Rates Reported in Academic Research and UK Mass Media." *International Journal of Men's Health* 14 (2). https://doi.org/10.3149/jmh.1402.86.

2 Parker, Lacie L., and Jennifer A. Harriger. 2020. "Eating Disorders and Disordered Eating Behaviors in the LGBT Population: A Review of the Literature." *Journal of Eating Disorders* 8 (1). https://doi.org/10.1186/s40337-020-00327-y.

3 Simone, Melissa, Vivienne M. Hazzard, Autumn J. Askew, Elliot A. Tebbe, Sarah K. Lipson, and Emily M. Pisetsky. 2022. "Variability in Eating Disorder Risk and Diagnosis in Transgender and Gender Diverse College Students." *Annals of Epidemiology* 70: 53–60. https://doi.org/10.1016/j.annepidem.2022.04.007.

4 Diemer, Elizabeth W., Julia D. Grant, Melissa A. Munn-Chernoff, David A. Patterson, and Alexis E. Duncan. 2015. "Gender Identity, Sexual Orientation, and Eating-Related Pathology in a National Sample of College Students." *Journal of Adolescent Health* 57 (2): 144–149. https://doi.org/10.1016/j.jadohealth.2015.03.003.

5 Samuels, Karen L., Margo M. Maine, and Mary Tantillo. 2019. "Disordered Eating, Eating Disorders, and Body Image in Midlife and Older Women." *Current Psychiatry Reports* 21 (8). https://doi.org/10.1007/s11920-019-1057-5.

6  Stewart, Lynn, Amy Usher, and Kim Allenby. 2009. *A Review of Optimal Group Size and Modularisation or Continuous Entry Format for Program Delivery*, June 2009, 1–20. www.csc-scc.gc.ca/005/008/092/005008-0215-01-eng.pdf.
7  Yalom, Irvin D., and Molyn Leszcz. 2005. *The Theory and Practice of Group Psychotherapy*. 5th ed. New York: Basic Books.
8  Strauss, Bernhard, Gary M. Burlingame, and Bianca Bormann. 2008. "Using the Core-R Battery in Group Psychotherapy." *Journal of Clinical Psychology* 64 (11): 1225–1237. https://doi.org/10.1002/jclp.20535.
9  Strauss et al., "Using the Core-R Battery," 1229.

# Appendix 2A: Provider Referral Form

## Provider Referral Form for Group

Date: _____

## Referring Provider Information:

Name: _____

Contact Information: _____

How long have you been working with this client? _____

## Client Information:

Name: _____

Briefly state why you think your client may benefit from the [Name] Group, particularly in relation to areas of concern regarding body image and their relationship with food.

_____

_____

Do you have any concerns regarding interpersonal dynamics? Please provide details, if applicable.

_____

_____

## Identified Diagnosis and Diagnosis Code:

Diagnosis: _____

Diagnosis Code: _____

### Family/Social Support and Psycho-social Information:

Please provide any relevant family/social support information or other psycho-social information that would assist in understanding the client's background and support network.

_____

_____

_____

### Progress Updates:

Would you like to receive updates on your client/patient's progress in the group? If so, please indicate your preferred method of communication (e.g., fax, phone call/message on voicemail) and frequency of updates.

_____

### Additional Information:

Is there anything else we need to know or that you believe would be helpful in working with your client?

_____

_____

Thank You!
Facilitators' Information:
Facilitator Name(s): _____
Contact Information: _____

# Appendix 2B: Group Application (For an Adult Group)

Thank you for requesting a [Name of Group] application. Please complete this application in its entirety and email the completed application back to [co-facilitators' names] at [email address] *or* fax to [fax number].

Name: _____ DOB: __/__/___ Age: _____
Phone Number: _____
Address:_____
Email: _____

Note: By providing your email address, you consent to us contacting you via this mode of communication.

Pronouns (circle): She/Her    He/Him    They/Them    Other
Briefly describe your eating disorder history:

_____
_____
_____
_____
_____

Have you received treatment for your eating disorder before other than an outpatient team? Please list any inpatient, residential, partial hospitalization program (PHP), or intensive outpatient (IOP) admissions and corresponding dates:

_____
_____
_____
_____

Describe the frequency of *current* symptom use:

Restricting: _____

Bingeing: _____

Purging: _____

Laxatives/Diuretics/Diet Pills: _____

Chewing/Spitting: _____

Excessive Exercise: _____

Body Checking:_____

Other: _____


What are some of your goals at this point in your recovery? What are you looking to get out of this group?

_____

_____

_____

Are there any specific topics or areas you want this group to cover?

_____

_____

_____

**Your Treatment Team:**

**Note:** Listing your treatment team providers is different from providing us with a release to contact them. We will only contact providers that you list if you sign a separate consent form for this provider. If you are uncomfortable listing your providers' names, please check the box to indicate that you regularly see this type of provider.

Therapist: _____

Dietitian: _____

Psychiatrist: _____

Family therapist: _____

Other: _____

Do you plan to get reimbursement for participation in this group from your insurance providers? (circle one) Y/N

Note: The group participation fee is $[fee] per session.

By signing below, I verify that all of the information on this form is truthful and that this application was completed by the person whose name is on this form.

Application Signature: _____    Date: _____

# Appendix 2C – Informed Consent (Sample Geared Toward a Group for Adult Women)

[Group Name]

## What to Expect

The group consists of both education and processing time. The experience will allow group members to give and receive support around body image, relationships with food and weight, diet culture, self-esteem, and other topics. The facilitators will use talk and experiential modalities to provide a rich and dynamic experience.

It is important to know that engaging in any form of therapy, including groups, can evoke discomfort, anxiety, and fear or trigger strong emotions such as anger and sadness; however, these emotions are often temporary and can lead to feelings of hope and positivity. Personal growth and change may be easy and swift at times but also may be slow and frustrating. Group members should address any concerns regarding progress with the facilitators.

The group dynamic offers a place to experience support, give support, and understand and improve group members' relationship with food and their bodies. Not only may members feel "not alone" in their struggles, but they will also feel supported in this process as they inspire and push each other to examine thoughts and ideas that may hold them back from living life and feeling good about themselves. These dynamics provide a compelling environment for change. Remember, the more group members give of themselves during the sessions, the more they will receive. The more honest and open group members are, the more space there is available for insight and growth.

The group experience is designed to complement individual therapy and should not be considered a substitute. If certain issues arise during the group process that are better addressed in individual therapy, facilitators may suggest that the member follow up with their individual therapist for further support. Furthermore, the facilitators may periodically communicate with the group member's outpatient therapist and, if applicable, their dietitian to provide updates on progress. A written authorization will be requested to obtain and receive information between the group facilitators and the relevant outpatient provider(s) to ensure a comprehensive and coordinated approach to the patient's treatment.

Group therapy is a powerful and valuable venue for healing and growth, and the group facilitators, [Facilitators' Names], are committed to creating an environment where members can experience the full benefits it offers. The facilitators strive to provide a confidential, recovery-focused space where every member feels respected and valued. They are dedicated to promoting a Health at Every Size® (HAES®) framework, rejecting diet culture, and challenging the notion that anything is "normal" or acceptable when it comes to the normative discontent women often experience about their bodies. The facilitators recognize the importance of fostering self-acceptance and a compassionate approach to oneself and others within the group.

## Attendance

Each member's presence in the group is important. Group dynamics are formed that help create an environment for growth and change. If group members are consistently absent, the group dynamic suffers. Therefore, facilitators ask that group members make this commitment a priority. It is understood that occasionally members may have to miss group due to an emergency, illness, vacation, or another important commitment (i.e. birthday dinner). If group members are unable to attend a group due to an emergency or illness, it is important for them to promptly contact the group facilitators prior to the scheduled group. To ensure effective communication, the preferred method of contact is email.

If group members know they will miss a future group, facilitators ask that this be relayed at least 24 hours in advance. This communication allows the facilitators to be informed in a timely manner and make any necessary adjustments or accommodations for the absence.

When group members leave, facilitators like to acknowledge this transition. Recognizing a participant's departure is done even if a member "pauses" their participation and rejoins at a later date. This acknowledgment aligns with the commitment to mutual support and the belief that everyone is important; their presence and absence impact group members and facilitators.

## Confidentiality

Group members must agree to maintain the confidentiality of other group members. Maintaining confidentiality means refraining from disclosing names or other identifying information about group members to anyone outside of the group; however, discussing your own experience of being in the group with non-members is acceptable.

Facilitators will protect the identity of each group participant by only allowing the use of first names and last initials within the group.

This group's policy is that group facilitators will not distribute the personal contact information of group participants. However, there are a few exceptions to confidentiality, including:

1. Active or suspected abuse (physical, emotional, or sexual) or neglect of a child, an elder, or a dependent adult must be reported to the appropriate protective service agency by [therapist's name].
2. If a group member threatens to harm herself or another individual, [therapist's name] is required to take steps to help maintain the safety of the person at risk.

## Telephone Accessibility and Emergencies

The group facilitators are unavailable via telephone or email for clinical or dietary support. They will monitor the [group name] email account (if applicable) for emails regarding logistics, absences, and other group-related inquiries. For clinical emergencies that require immediate attention or action, they will need to call 911, [name and number of local crisis resources], or go to the nearest emergency room.

## Professional Fees and Payment

The total cost of this group is $[fee] for each [time]-minute group session. Group members are required to keep valid credit card information on file. Unless otherwise agreed upon, this credit card will only be used for group sessions and charged following each session.

## Insurance and Managed Care

For group members who plan to file for reimbursement (typically using an out-of-network benefit) through their insurance company, a detailed statement that contains provider information and their relevant diagnostic code(s) will be provided via email after the group. It is important to have thoroughly reviewed and understand the insurance company's reimbursement policies, the amount of their deductible, the percentage their company will reimburse for outpatient group psychotherapy, and any limitations to treatment that may be a stipulation of their policy. The contract for reimbursement is between the insurance holder and their insurance company rather than between the insurance company and the group facilitators.

I have read the Informed Consent Agreement for the [Name] Group. My signature on this form shows that I understand the information and agree to the terms of group participation.

Signature: _____

Printed Name: _____

Date: _____

# Chapter 3

# Strategies for a Successful Group

## Enhancing Design, Facilitation, and Evaluation in Group Therapy

Group facilitators have the potential to design a group culture of support and connection. This chapter provides practical guidance for Registered Dietitians and therapists facilitating outpatient eating disorder group therapy, focusing on enhancing efficiency and effectiveness. It emphasizes the importance of creating a safe and supportive group culture, with facilitators playing a key role in setting the tone through attunement, emotional regulation, and establishing clear rules and boundaries.

This chapter is split into five parts. The chapter begins with part one, highlighting the benefits of mixed-diagnosis groups and exploring different group modalities. Part two focuses on equipping facilitators with essential skills for successful group leadership. It emphasizes the significance of appropriate time management, as it enhances group dynamics and encourages active participant involvement. Part three covers the establishment of clear rules and boundaries. By defining and effectively communicating these guidelines, facilitators enable group members to understand their roles and responsibilities in fostering a more cohesive and productive environment. Part four delves into common challenges that may arise within the group and provides practical suggestions for troubleshooting. Conflicts, communication breakdowns, and lack of participation are addressed, offering strategies to overcome these obstacles and promote positive group dynamics. It covers providing effective feedback to participants, recognizing their strengths, and identifying areas where additional support or referral to a higher level of care may be required. Lastly, part five addresses group evaluations. By gathering feedback and monitoring the effectiveness of the group, facilitators can make necessary adjustments and continuously improve the group experience.

By addressing these key aspects, facilitators can create and maintain a supportive and impactful group experience for themselves and the participants. The insights shared in this chapter aim to empower facilitators and enhance the overall effectiveness of group facilitation.

DOI: 10.4324/9781003430964-5

## Part One

### Understanding Diagnoses

The most common eating disorders based on the Diagnostic and Statistical Manual of Mental Disorders, 5th edition (DSM-5), include Anorexia Nervosa (AN), Bulimia Nervosa (BN), Binge-Eating Disorder (BED), Avoidant and Restrictive Food Intake Disorder (ARFID), Other Specified Feeding and Eating Disorder (OSFED), and Unspecified Feeding or Eating Disorder (USFED), with the latter being a preliminary diagnosis used when eating disorder behaviors are present but there is insufficient information to make a firm diagnosis.

Common factors contributing to the persistence of BN, AN, and other eating disorders include perfectionism, core low self-esteem, mood intolerance, and interpersonal difficulties.[1] Body image disturbances transcend diagnosis (except ARFID), as does weight stigma. The symptoms of eating disorders result from complex interactions between biological, psychological, and social factors.

Eating disorders exist on a continuum, encompassing a range of symptom acuity and diverse symptom presentations. It is common for individuals to transition over time, moving from restrictive eating patterns to episodes of binge eating and potentially incorporating purging behaviors such as self-induced vomiting, excessive exercise, or laxative abuse.

A person's experiences or behaviors do not need to change dramatically to warrant a change in diagnosis. For example, a person diagnosed with Anorexia Nervosa, binge-purge subtype, who gains sufficient weight will garner a new diagnosis of Bulimia Nervosa and vice versa.

Diagnostic criteria are based on identifying positive symptoms over a three-month period, but the frequent fluctuations in weight and changes in symptoms mean that it is not unusual for individuals to have a high degree of crossover in their diagnoses.[2] This crossover is one challenge of a homogeneous diagnosis group because members can and do frequently change diagnoses across the eating disorder spectrum. Considering the potential for diagnostic crossover, it is important to create an inclusive and flexible group approach that acknowledges the dynamic nature of eating disorders and accommodates individuals with diverse symptom presentations.

Group facilitators are encouraged to avoid using specific diagnostic labels in the group setting and instead use the term "eating disorders." Aside from the high degree of crossover in diagnoses, this recommendation is an effort to challenge the belief in a diagnostic hierarchy. A belief among individuals with eating disorders, the general population, and even some medical professionals hold that eating disorder acuity is hierarchical, with AN typical at the top and BED at the bottom. As stated by researcher Rose Mortimer, "despite significant similarities between the various different eating disorders, they are often conceived of in binary terms: chaos and control; disgust and purity; vice and virtue."[3]

The focus should be on understanding and addressing the underlying issues and shared experiences related to eating disorders rather than categorizing individuals based on specific diagnoses. Most theoretical models of eating disorders posit that emotions are often poorly regulated and that individuals with eating disorders often turn to food or control their weight, shape, or size to manage and regulate their emotions.[4] Regardless of their eating disorder diagnosis, there is a universality in their emotional suffering and the desire for relief from that suffering. This shared experience across diagnoses enables members to relate, connect, and enrich each other's recovery.

### To Mix or Not to Mix?

Some clinicians shy away from a mixed-diagnosis group because they worry that group members will feel like they cannot relate to one another. This is far from the truth. Mixed-diagnosis groups certainly have their benefits and drawbacks, and sometimes these challenges benefit the group.

In a mixed-diagnosis group, the presence of diverse body shapes and sizes can evoke fear of judgment among members. However, this diversity also presents an opportunity to confront weight bias and the fear of rejection perpetuating eating disorders. Individuals in larger bodies may feel self-conscious when smaller-bodied members express dissatisfaction with their weight or shape. Similarly, those struggling with a fear of weight gain may encounter a group member who embodies their feared body type. These encounters compel individuals to confront their internalized weight stigma. It is important to foster discussions about weight stigma and thin privilege, encouraging members to examine the meaning attributed to physical bodies and challenging their acceptance of societal beliefs. Further exploration of weight stigma and thin privilege will be covered in Chapter 8.

Individuals in larger bodies can derive benefit from witnessing that weight loss does not guarantee happiness or self-worth. Many of them may have experienced being in smaller bodies. They can share their insights on how body shape or size did not correlate with emotional or physical well-being. This perspective challenges the notion that thinness inherently equates to a better quality of life and helps dismantle harmful societal beliefs surrounding body image.

Research offers valuable insights into the complex nature and course of clinical eating disorders, providing a deeper understanding of the entire spectrum. A perspective emerges that emphasizes shared experiences and commonalities, which may overshadow any discomfort arising from differences. The study authors emphasize that the frequent movement of patients between various diagnoses strengthens the notion that these disorders share important similarities, suggesting that they could be viewed as a single entity.[5] We firmly believe that by employing skilled group facilitation and adopting a collaborative approach, the shared experiences and commonalities will eclipse the discomfort that may arise from these differences.

### Group Modalities

Typically, eating disorder groups use a specific format such as process, psychoeducation, multi-family, or support. They also may focus on specific modalities such as Cognitive Behavioral Therapy [CBT], Interpersonal Psychotherapy [ITP], or Dialectical Behavioral Therapy [DBT]. We have found that using an amalgamation of modalities and formats effectively engages different learning and processing styles.

We use various experiential interventions because traditional talk therapy, even evidenced-based therapies for treating eating disorders like CBT, falls short when trying to help group members identify and release the pain that keeps them stuck in behaviors they know are harmful. These interventions include guided imagery, meditations, role-playing exercises, expressive writing, art-based activities (like collage), photography exploration, and mindful eating exercises. Experiential interventions allow members to break through the defenses the eating disorder hides behind. It also allows a felt experience in the present that is necessary for insight and movement toward full recovery.

## Part Two

### Skills for Leading Group

Running an effective group requires a balance between process and content. Process refers to how information is managed, including interactions and relationships among members within the group. Content refers to the information shared.[6] In their research on group work, Geroski and Kraus interviewed scholars in the field regarding content and process. One scholar likened the process to a river and content to a boat on the river.[7]

When group facilitators solely focus on imparting information (content) without attuning to the group dynamics, it can negatively impact the members' engagement and participation. For instance, if a dietitian provides education on nutritional science to challenge eating disorder rules or a therapist teaches the skill of mindfulness without considering the group's dynamics, members may feel their individual experiences and emotions are not acknowledged or validated. This experience of invalidation can lead to their withdrawal from the group, both mentally and physically, as they may perceive the group as an environment where they are not truly seen or understood. Group facilitators must balance delivering content and fostering a supportive and attuned environment that encourages active participation and validates group members' experiences. Integrating an awareness of group dynamics and individual emotional needs into their approach allows facilitators to create a more inclusive and enriching group experience where members feel seen, heard, and valued. Conversely, if the attention is focused only on the eliciting emotions (process), members may question what they learned and why they joined the group in the first place.

We integrate content and process by eliciting feedback and utilizing co-facilitation. We recommend obtaining feedback regarding the group experience to ensure that the group is balanced to meet members' needs. Feedback may be obtained by emailing out a survey or having a discussion during a group. As referenced in Chapter 1, co-facilitation allows a group facilitator to drive a discussion. At the same time, the other facilitator can be more attuned to group dynamics to include members' responses and needs as they learn new skills, gain insights, and feel seen, heard, and supported. The goal is for members to feel like they are learning and growing.

### Why is Group Therapy Hard for Facilitators?

Despite careful recruitment and assessment of group members, it is important to recognize that they are still a group of individuals with varying levels of needs, attachment histories, and emotional health. The members and the facilitators themselves are bound to experience some degree of affective dysregulation due to the intensity of group work. When facilitators meet these challenges with empathy and compassion for themselves and the group members, the group has the potential to become a transformative haven in recovery.

*Building Empathy*

As clinicians specializing in treating eating disorders, we support our patients and their loved ones in understanding the drivers of their symptoms. Typically those drivers are related to emotional pain, such as feelings of worthlessness or abandonment. Seeing these connections allows loved ones to access empathy and validation and for the patients to access self-compassion. Identification of these drivers is also an opportunity to address underlying needs.

We ask the same of ourselves as eating disorder clinicians. Looking at challenging group members' behavior with curiosity and compassion can help the facilitators remain regulated and select interventions that are sensitive to the members' experiences and needs. Reflecting on one's transference or counter-transference is critical.

For those who struggle with social anxiety and attachment-related fear of judgment or rejection, the group may allow for a corrective experience. Others may fear reenacting relational ruptures and become confrontational, dismissive, or withdrawn as a protective defense. It is important to be aware of transference and projection that members may be responding and reacting to and have compassion for that member's experience. Accessing that compassion can be especially difficult when the group facilitators or other group members are the objects of negative transference.

### Staying Regulated

The responsibilities of group facilitators are to attend to group members by imparting information, guiding interpersonal interactions, and keeping the space emotionally safe. Even for the most skilled practitioners, this can feel daunting. There are many eyes on the group facilitators. It follows that when the facilitator inevitably misses a cue or a topic falls flat, as evidenced by silence or resistance, it can activate the clinician's threat system. The facilitator may notice sweat under their armpits, their face getting warm, or paralysis leaving them at a loss for what to say next. They should slow down and take a few deep belly breaths. Taking a sip of water and feeling their feet on the floor and their bottom on their chair are ways to ground and give themselves compassion.

It is important to reflect on how facilitators feel about their group members. Facilitators may become the subject of a member's transference, leading to countertransference. Having a co-facilitator and allocating time for debriefing after the group can be advantageous in addressing these dynamics. Sharing frustration or hearing a different account of how their partner experienced the group can be validating and insightful for their growth as a clinician.

### Facilitation Tips

While the role of the group facilitator is one of great responsibility, a sure-fire way to burn out as a group leader is doing for the group what the group can do for itself. Encourage group members to support and encourage one another. This encouragement can be done by modeling these skills, furthering members to check in with each other, and asking members periodically for feedback on topics and group structure to increase investment and engagement.

Just like members can present with challenging behaviors that potentially compromise the efficacy of the group process, group facilitators' behaviors have the same potential.

We suggest the following:

- Encourage members to test the waters, gradually open up and share their experiences as they develop a sense of safety within the group rather than pressuring them to disclose information prematurely.
- Intervene promptly when potentially harmful experiences, such as aggression or humiliation, occur in the group setting.
- Remember not to impose personal values on group members, respecting their unique perspectives and experiences.

- Provide a supportive and structured environment while remaining flexible regarding the agenda and procedures to accommodate the members' needs.
- Avoid rescuing members who express distress by changing the topic or excessively focusing on their distress. Instead, offer validation and empathy as powerful interventions.
- Remember that facilitators do not need to have all the answers. Validation and empathy are the most powerful interventions.

### Time Allocation (Prep, In-Group, and Debriefing)

Time allocation is an important consideration for the direct time spent in the group as well as indirect time spent outside of the group. Preparation before a series of closed group sessions or to prepare for ongoing groups with a rolling admission is vital to the efficacy of the group's interventions. Facilitators should set aside a predetermined amount of time before the group to review anticipated attendance, choose a specific group discussion or activity, and determine how much time to allocate to those activities (i.e., check-in and experiential activity). Facilitators must remain flexible with their plans to ensure they can be responsive to the group's needs. For example, suppose body image is a theme among several members' check-ins. In that case, facilitators may pivot to a different activity related to body image than the one they had planned.

After either an in-person or virtual group, a debriefing between facilitators allows them to share any notable clinical impressions of individual members or group dynamics. This consultation may inform interventions for the following group or trigger a call or email to the individual's dietitian, therapist, or member to discuss concerns. Depending on how billing is handled, members may require facilitators to provide superbills or submit insurance claims for the group, so time should also be allocated for these responsibilities.

## Part Three

### Rules and Boundaries

Group rules can be conceptualized as codes of conduct or guidelines intended to reduce members' anxieties and promote therapeutic norms. As referenced in Chapter 2, group members will be given an Informed Consent document before participating in the group. In addition to information on the group's attendance policy, confidentiality, fees, and payment, the Informed Consent also includes the group's rules and boundaries.

For closed fixed-session groups, we recommend reviewing group rules with the group members early in the first session. In an ongoing, closed group with rolling admission, we encourage the review of group rules whenever a new member begins. In our group, each time a new member joins, the members share the group's ground rules and give examples to the new member. It provides the new member with this information and serves as a refresher for current members. It may even spur a discussion, such as how the group's rules compare to groups they may have been in in the past or defining some vague terms like "triggering." We also encourage members to create or adjust guidelines, with the facilitators' support, in response to issues that may arise within the group.

Group guidelines or rules can be written in various ways, such as using pronouns "I" or "We" or simply laying out expectations with or without rationale included (although it is recommended the rationale is explained). The following are the most commonly recommended group rules and their rationales:

*Table 3.1* Sample group rules/guidelines with accompanying rationale.

| Group Rule/Guideline | Rationale |
| --- | --- |
| Respect and maintain the confidentiality of group members. This confidentiality includes names and any other identifying characteristics of group members. | Having clear guidelines about confidentiality protects members' privacy and increases comfort in self-disclosure. |
| Speak from your own experiences instead of generalizing ("I/They" instead of "we" and "you"). | Speaking for yourself minimizes misunderstanding, misrepresentation, and invalidation. It allows members to practice being assertive and taking ownership of their stories. |
| Participate to the fullest of your ability. | The pace at which a member builds trust to allow vulnerability varies. Community growth depends on the inclusion of every individual voice. |
| Give supportive attention to the person who is speaking and avoid side conversations. | Active listening fosters an attunement where members feel valued. |
| Refrain from discussing group members who are not present. | Members who are no longer in the group or unable to attend a session cannot speak for themselves. Discussions about absent members can undermine trust in the group. |
| Members may ask each other direct questions but choose not to answer if they are uncomfortable or feel unprepared to share information with the group. | This rule encourages members to demonstrate genuine interest and care toward each other while emphasizing the importance of setting and respecting personal boundaries. |
| Refrain from using specific numbers regarding weight, nutritional information, and exercise. Members can identify symptoms, for example: purging, restricting, and bingeing. | Numbers can trigger eating disorder thoughts; specifically, they promote comparison, may glorify symptoms, and are unnecessary to convey a message. |

| Group Rule/Guideline | Rationale |
|---|---|
| Be respectful and accepting of the diversity of people's experiences and feelings. | By emphasizing the importance of respecting diversity, this group rule promotes emotional safety and encourages an accepting environment for everyone's experiences and feelings. |
| Attend groups on time. Members are asked to prioritize the group by attending all sessions, arriving on time, and remaining for the entire session. Members who cannot attend a session are expected to contact a facilitator at least 24 hours beforehand. | Attending a group consistently and showing up on time shows investment in the group and respect for fellow members. Providing ample notice allows group leaders to adjust the agenda for the group or cancel the group if the census is too low to conduct an effective group. |

## Part Four

### Managing Common Problems and Challenges

The group dynamic offers a place to experience and give support, understand, and improve group members' relationship with food and their body. We hope members will feel supported in this process as they inspire and push each other to examine thoughts and ideas that may hold them back from living life, feel less alone in their struggles, and feel good about themselves. These dynamics provide a powerful environment for change.

It would be unrealistic to expect all group members to demonstrate the same level of participation, compassion, and attunement. When there are significant outliers to group norms, these deteriorate group cohesion. While not always readily apparent, the roots of conflict within the group can often be traced back to significant challenges individuals face. When group members exhibit behaviors challenging group norms, it is the facilitators' responsibility to address them skillfully. The norms help others know what to expect and set the stage for attachment security.

There are a host of reasons group therapy can be challenging for members. Members have shared fearing they will "say the wrong thing," look foolish, or not be liked. They may worry they are not sick enough or too sick. Some need help sharing the group facilitator's attention with the other members, which can be especially challenging if the group facilitators work with member(s) individually. For these types of group concerns, Discussion 4.1 is a great resource.

### Interpersonal Conflict Within Group

The types of conflict we generally see in our groups are not typically loud or hostile. More often they are subtle, expressed by body language; for example, an eye roll, a change in tone of voice, or a change in the level of participation. A misunderstanding usually triggers the conflict, be it a misinterpretation of the leader's or a member's body language, disclosure, or feedback.

As group facilitators, we try to stay attuned to these subtle signs of a conflict brewing and address them in the moment by sharing our observations and furthering members to clarify what they heard the facilitator or member say. This technique allows for practicing assertive communication and curtailing the escalation of a conflict. It also provides an increased understanding of themselves and each other, which builds cohesion and connection. If the group facilitators manage challenging behaviors skillfully, the chances of conflicts arising are reduced.

## Common Group Disruptions

The following are the most common group disruptions we encounter and suggestions for handling them.

### Coming Late/Missing Groups

Tardiness or repeatedly missing the group can be framed as an attachment rupture as it threatens members' emotional safety.

For some members, this may support the narrative that they are not important and not worth the investment of others. Members being chronically late or absent threatens the cohesion of the group. It can lead to feelings of disconnection or resentment by members (and even facilitators) who show a higher level of commitment by consistently showing up for each group on time.

Recommended Interventions:

- Inquire about this behavior with curiosity, reserving judgment. Members may already feel shame for lateness or missing a group.
- Review group rules carefully before the group, at the start of the group, or by email after the group.
- If it is one person consistently, discuss individually with that member what may be barriers to attending or being on time. Help problem solve if indicated.

### Silence and Lack of Participation

A group's success depends on the level of interaction among group members. Members who are silent or consistently share only minimally impact the entire group. Other group members sharing more consistently may become self-conscious and begin to feel they are talking too much and become quiet. Other members may feel the burden to keep the conversation going. Feelings of disconnection and even resentment may develop.

There are many reasons group members may be silent or speak minimally. Sometimes it is as simple as needing clarification on how the group process works, specifically the protocol for sharing. Members may be used to a classroom or meeting structure and are waiting to be called on by a group leader. Members may believe they have nothing to add to the discussion or fear inadvertently offending or triggering other members. They may not be used to talking about themselves and have gotten messages that doing so is selfish or vain. They may feel their problems are less severe than their peers and feel foolish asking for support. Lastly, members lacking the trust of others and fearing rejection may feel safer as an observer, at least until they are more familiar with the group culture.

Recommended Interventions:

- Structure the group's activities to give room for every member to participate.
- Ask open-ended questions specific to individual members.
- Give them room to share opinions and insights, including asking specifically for this member's input.
- Use ice breakers (see Chapter 4).
- Assign group members homework.

### Monopolistic Behavior

Members with monopolistic behavior appear to take over the group by continuously bringing things back to themselves. They lack attunement to the needs of other group members and in some cases miss social cues. Monopolizing could take the form of storytelling, where the member provides details that do not add value and are unnecessary to receive support. The member's thought process is typically circumstantial and can even be tangential. This takes time; other members lose interest or become confused and frustrated.

The causal factors for monopolistic behaviors vary. As mentioned earlier, members may feel compelled to keep talking if other members are not talking or sharing. Their discomfort with the disturbances in their thought process or their lack of awareness of social cues may be related to comorbidities including but not limited to Obsessive Compulsive Disorder, Anxiety Disorders, Autistic Spectrum Disorders, or a traumatic brain injury.

Recommended Interventions:

- Summarize main points and redirect
- Show appreciation for their willingness to share and indicate a desire to ensure that others also have an opportunity to contribute.
- Emphasize that stories should focus on how the event made them feel rather than each detail.
- Ask the group for input, encouraging others to contribute.
- Ask explicitly to hear from other group members.
- Ask this individual to pause to create space for others to process and share.

### Demanding Attention and Validation from the Group Facilitator(s)

When members share their experiences in the group, many express a desire for support from individuals who can truly relate to their struggles, wanting support from people who are "in it." While they may appreciate the feedback, validation, and empathy therapists or dietitians provide, there is something about getting support from peers that is extremely powerful and can even have a legitimacy to them that practitioners may lack. In our experience, the most effective groups are those where we introduce a topic, provide psychoeducation or activity, and then step back, allowing members to engage in meaningful conversations with one another.

Nevertheless, some members consistently seek direct feedback from the group facilitators rather than from other group members. This dynamic can be complex, particularly if the group facilitator also serves as a member's therapist or dietitian. They may feel more comfortable in this dynamic and may not trust the members to understand them the way they perceive the facilitators will. Therefore, we encourage facilitators to foster an atmosphere that urges members to utilize the group for support rather than relying solely on individual interactions with the facilitators.

Recommended Interventions:

- Redirect questions to the group by asking the group members to share their thoughts.
- Sensitively point out this pattern during the group or 1:1 with curiosity and encouragement to utilize the group.

### Help Rejecting Complainers (HRC)

In 1952, psychiatrist Jerome Frank coined the term help-rejecting complainer to describe an individual who complains in order to seek advice and help, only to reject it.[8] In the group, this member seeks the group facilitators' or the group members' attention by implicitly or explicitly asking for help and then rejecting any help offered. The problems sound impossible to solve, and some pride may be taken in how hopeless their situation appears. The member may overtly or subtly belittle the problems of others, and at times other group members may belittle their own problems in response to this member. The member may blame others for their problems or have difficulty accepting personal responsibility or accountability. The lack of personal accountability prevents them from feeling empowered to make a change. This presentation also monopolizes the group members' and facilitators' time and energy.

Recommended Interventions:

- Avoid showing anger and frustration because they maintain HRC's belief that no one understands them.
- Redirect members who offer advice because it will typically maintain the cycle.
- Provide empathy and ask what their plan is to address this problem.
- Ask what type of support they want from the group
- Use empathy and share the experience of help rejection, including how that impacts group members and the facilitators.
- Do not continue to offer help outside of validation and empathy.

### Advice Giving

Members may feel pressure to "fix" the problems presented by group members and take up the role of an advice-giver. Advice giving may look like telling members what they should do or how they should or should not feel. These members may see themselves as further along in recovery and may be further along in recovery. They might feel they know how to overcome other group members' challenges, but the advice may not be sound. While there may be times when a member would like feedback in the form of suggestions from group members, it is recommended that members clarify if they want suggestions or help with problem-solving. Often, we find that people just want to feel heard.

Recommended Interventions:

- When members share a problem, model active listening and ask questions. Encourage other members to do the same.
- Group members can share insight and tell what has worked for them.
- Encourage members to indicate if they want suggestions or help with problem-solving.

### Rescuing

Rescuing behavior includes rushing in to comfort another who is upset and supplying the answer for another who is struggling to find one for themselves. The rescuers appear to wish to help the other yet are often motivated by their need to reduce their anxiety or distress triggered by seeing another person's discomfort. Members may have developed the tendency to rescue in response to a family culture where showing emotional distress was not tolerated or where they felt responsible for regulating the emotions of others. They may see their value coming from what they can give to others. Jokes and changing the subject can also be rescuing behavior. While this group member may be trying to be supportive, the effect is shutting down uncomfortable emotions, perpetuating the notion that those emotions are dangerous and must be avoided.

Recommended Interventions:

- With sensitivity, invite the rescuer to focus their attention on themselves and the rescuing behavior.
- In sharing this observation, ask other members if they can relate.

- Use this as a group topic, framing it as a role they felt compelled to take for survival that is no longer needed or workable.
- Encourage members to take on a monitoring role to kindly "call out" this behavior.
- Encourage members to make space for all their emotions that arise compassionately and non-judgmentally.

### When Outpatient Group Therapy is Not a Good Fit or Not Enough

Ideally, members of an outpatient group would be appropriate for outpatient care, but this is not always the case. For one, selection errors occur. These commonly result in a mismatch between the therapeutic modality – in this case the group – and the acuity of the member's psychopathology. For instance, a member with Schizoid or Avoidant Personality traits may struggle with the interpersonal functioning required to interact in such a complex system. Others may be, or at least appear, appropriate at the start, but changes in symptomatology may require a re-evaluation of their appropriateness for care in the outpatient group setting. While this is not an exhaustive list, some red flags that indicate the need for a higher level of care or alternative treatment include:

- Inability to refrain from movement or exercise while in the group (i.e., engaging in isometric exercise)
- Psychomotor retardation or agitation
- Glorification of the eating disorder; difficulty identifying reasons to recover or negative consequences of their eating disorder for themself or others
- Report of an uptick in symptom use without or with limited support, skills, or motivation to change
- Preoccupation with intrusive, repetitive thoughts (surmised by the need for constant redirection in the group)

Co-facilitators should discuss concerns related to members' appropriateness for the group. The members depend on the facilitators to maintain a safe environment. Our experience is that our members have shared concern for others when they see these "red flags." They may feel helpless and look to the facilitators to unburden them from their concerns.

While we encourage group members to share their concerns directly with each other, they may worry about how their concerns will be received. Even if the concerns are addressed during group, it may warrant the facilitators meeting with the member individually to discuss whether a different level of care may be more appropriate. This recommendation should always be made with ample communication with this member's outpatient team.

We encourage members to communicate directly to the group or write a message to the group (which the facilitators can read) if the member is seeking more intensive care or leaving the group.

## Part Five

### Group Evaluations

As facilitators, we are committed to providing groups that meet our members' needs. If we do not, members will not show improvement in treatment outcomes and may, understandably, drop out of the group. Not meeting our members' needs may even lead to adverse outcomes for an individual member or the group as a whole. To effectively identify and improve the treatment experience, eliciting feedback from group members is vital. We cannot depend on our observations alone to assess members' experiences of group therapy or the efficacy of the treatment.

Encouraging members to provide feedback to the facilitators underscores the transformative power of the group itself as a change agent. The active involvement and feedback from group members and the facilitators' responsiveness contribute to the group's dynamic and collaborative environment.

Depending on the type of group – closed fixed-session or open with rolling admission, virtual or in-person – the timing of an evaluation and the specific questions asked will vary. For example, for a group on a six-week session cycle, a questionnaire may be given after they have completed all six sessions. For an in-person group, there may be questions about the comfort of the physical environment. For a virtual group, questions may relate to the virtual platform's ease of use. A sample of this type of evaluation is provided in Appendix 3A. For ongoing, rolling admission groups, leaving members may be asked to complete a questionnaire evaluating the group after their last group. Active participants may be asked periodically to provide feedback via a written questionnaire or asked individually. A sample questionnaire for enrolled group members is provided in Appendix 3B.

Eliciting feedback can be incorporated into a group activity. It requires vulnerability and self-reflection. It provides an opportunity to practice interpersonal communication skills like assertiveness. It may also increase members' sense of agency and community.

It is recommended that group facilitators evaluate periodically to understand the experience of group members better and make the necessary adjustments based on this feedback. For an example of group evaluations, see the Sample Group Evaluation for a Fixed-Session Group (Appendix 3A) and the Sample Group Evaluation for an Ongoing, Rolling Admission Group (Appendix 3B).

## Notes

1 Cooper, Zafra, and Riccardo Dalle Grave. "Chapter 14 – Eating Disorders: Transdiagnostic Theory and Treatment." In *The Science of Cognitive Behavioral Therapy*, edited by Stefan G. Hofmann and Gordon J. G. Asmundson. Cambridge, MA: Academic Press. 337–357.
2 Mortimer, Rose. 2019. "Pride before a Fall: Shame, Diagnostic Crossover, and Eating Disorders." *Journal of Bioethical Inquiry* 16 (3): 365–374. https://doi.org/10.1007/s11673-019-09923-3.
3 Mortimer, "Pride before a Fall," 366.
4 Henderson, Ziporah B., John R. E. Fox, Penny Trayner, and Anja Wittkowski. 2019. "Emotional Development in Eating Disorders: A Qualitative Metasynthesis." *Clinical Psychology & Psychotherapy* 26 (4): 440–457. https://doi.org/10.1002/cpp.2365.
5 Milos, Gabriella, Anja Spindler, Ulrich Schnyder, and Christopher G. Fairburn. 2005. "Instability of Eating Disorder Diagnoses: Prospective Study." *The British Journal of Psychiatry* 187 (6): 573–578. https://doi.org/10.1192/bjp.187.6.573.
6 Gladding, Samuel T., and Mark A. Binkley. 2007. *Advancing Groups: Practical Ways Leaders Can Work Through Some Problematic Situations* (ACAPCD-11). Alexandria, VA: American Counseling Association.
7 Geroski, Anne, and Kurt Kraus. 2002. "Process and Content in School Psychoeducational Groups:" *The Journal for Specialists in Group Work* 27 (2): 233–245. https://doi.org/10.1080/742848694.
8 Frank, Jerome D., Eduard Ascher, Joseph B. Margolin, Helen Nash, Anthony R. Stone, and Edith J. Varon. 1952. "Behavioral Patterns in Early Meetings of Therapeutic Groups." *American Journal of Psychiatry* 108 (10): 771–778. https://doi.org/10.1176/ajp.108.10.771.

# Appendix 3A: Sample Group Evaluation for a Fixed-Session Group

The following evaluation is a sample for a six-week, 75-minute group.

## Group Evaluation Questionnaire

We value your feedback and suggestions as we continue to build, grow, and improve this group. Please take time to thoughtfully fill out this evaluation so that we can make the group even better.

Please rank the top three most beneficial topics from the following weekly themes. (Place a 1 in the box beside the most beneficial theme, a 2 beside the second . . .) If none were helpful, please leave this question blank.

[ ] Week 1, Taking Care of Myself Without the Eating Disorder
[ ] Week 2, Identity & Values
[ ] Week 3, Creating Change
[ ] Week 4, Social Justice and Diet Culture
[ ] Week 5, The Embodied Experience
[ ] Week 6, It All Comes Back to the Food

2. Are there any specific *themes or topics* you wish were covered?

_____

_____

_____

3. Are there any specific *modalities* you wish were included (i.e., role-playing, expressive/art, psychodrama, etc.)?

_____

_____

_____

4. Did you have a favorite part of the group?

_____

_____

_____

5. What is one thing you would change about this group?

_____

_____

_____

6. Was the six-week cycle too short? Too long? Just right? Did 75 minutes feel like enough time for the group?

_____

_____

_____

7. Would you be interested in participating in another cycle of the group? YES NO (circle one)

If yes, what would you like to see covered? How would you like it to be different from this cycle?

_____

_____

_____

8. Our goal is to create an environment where members feel safe being vulnerable and feel connected to the group while also feeling seen and valued individually. Please share any suggestions for how we can do this better.

_____

_____

_____

9. Is there anything else you would like us to know?

_____

_____

_____

Thank you for your time and participation.

# Appendix 3B: Sample Group Evaluation for an Ongoing, Rolling Admission Group

The following evaluation is a sample for an ongoing group. The evaluation could be used intermittently throughout members' participation in the group.

Are you satisfied with the group's time, duration, and frequency? If not, please provide alternative suggestions.

_____

_____

How is the group helping you reach your recovery goals? If it is not, do you have any suggestions regarding how the group can be more effective and useful?

_____

_____

Which previously covered topics would you like to revisit in future groups?

_____

_____

Identify topics or activities you would like to see in future groups.

_____

_____

Please check all activities/interventions that interest you:

☐ Guided imagery/Meditation
☐ Music
☐ Art
☐ Psychodrama
☐ Movement
☐ Book club
☐ Movies or video clips with discussion

☐   Exposures (food, body image)
☐   Other:

What changes or improvements do you think could enhance the group's physical or virtual environment?

_____

_____

Are there group rules or guidelines you feel need to be reinforced or revised?

_____

_____

What would you like the group facilitators to do more or less of to enhance your group experience?

_____

_____

Is there anything else you want us to know?

_____

_____

Thank you for your time and participation.

# Part II

# Chapter 4

# Building Community

## Cultivating Support and Connection in Eating Disorder Group Therapy

This chapter serves as a gateway to the book's second part, bridging the gap between the fundamentals of running an outpatient group and specific guidance on group content. It delves into the transformative power of the group community, emphasizing the necessity of group cohesion and providing effective strategies for building it.

As facilitators, our responsibility is to create a safe, non-judgmental, and emotionally inviting space conducive to healing and growth. This chapter explores intentional choices regarding group composition, structure, and physical and virtual environments that optimize the group's ability to engage in meaningful conversations, establish connections, and foster bonding and community.

We recognize the importance of openness and vulnerability in the group setting. This chapter introduces engaging discussions and a range of activities specifically designed to promote these qualities among group members. Through activities rooted in approaches such as narrative therapy, expressive therapy, and positive psychology, we aim to cultivate an environment where individuals can authentically share their experiences, thoughts, and emotions. These activities catalyze deepening connections and building a robust sense of community.

Practical guidance on seamlessly integrating new members into an established group is provided, enabling new participants to feel welcomed and valued. Furthermore, we address the process of bidding farewell to group members departing and offering termination rituals to promote a positive ending that honors their journey and contributions.

By implementing these activities and strategies, facilitators can nurture an environment conducive to trust, genuine sharing, and profound connections within the group community. Integrating Cognitive-Behavioral Therapy (CBT) techniques, psychoeducation, and Positive Psychology principles further enhances the therapeutic impact of the group experience.

As facilitators, we have witnessed the transformative power of a strong and supportive community, creating a space where individuals can find solace,

DOI: 10.4324/9781003430964-7

support, and inspiration as they navigate their unique paths toward healing and recovery.

## The Power of the Group Community

While higher levels of care often prioritize group therapy as a primary treatment modality, outpatient treatment traditionally revolves around appointments with an individual therapist, a family therapist, a dietitian, a psychiatrist, and a physician. Although outpatient groups are gaining recognition for their transformative and profound impact on recovery, it remains a fact that most individuals with eating disorders are not currently engaged in outpatient group therapy.

When out in "the real world," many members feel alone in their struggle with food. They may also feel alone in their efforts to disengage from talking about diets and hating their appearance. The group setting provides an opportunity for interpersonal growth that individual treatment cannot replicate. It provides a sense of belonging and mutual support, referred to as cohesion. Research has shown that finding others suffering similarly to their own nurtures a feeling of acceptance and belonging.[1] This shared experience facilitates vulnerability that group members may feel less inclined to have with a provider who might not have this same lived experience.

According to a 2017 meta-analysis of group psychotherapy for eating disorders published in the *International Journal of Eating Disorders*, group psychotherapy looks to be as effective as other common treatments and more cost-effective than individual therapy.[2] While we do not see the group modality as a replacement for individual therapy, it is a supplement with the potential to reinforce strides made in individual therapy and enrich treatment.

Clinicians reading this book understand the critical need to establish rapport with their patients. A wealth of research continuously shows the correlation between the quality of the relationship between therapist and patient with therapy outcomes.[3] In group therapy, however, these interactions are far more complex. There are multiple systems of interpersonal relationships and interactions happening simultaneously. Members have relationships with other members, the group as a whole, and the group facilitators. The facilitators have relationships with the members individually, the group as a whole, and their co-facilitator. The quality of all these relationships greatly affects the efficacy and success of the group.[4] This rapport does not happen overnight and can take considerable effort, reflection, and thought on the facilitators' behalf.

Consider that many people exhibiting an eating disorder or related symptoms feel a great deal of shame around these symptoms. They know that bingeing and purging are unhealthy for their bodies, yet the temporary relief makes it difficult to change their behavior. They know that food restriction can negatively impact every organ and system in their body, yet eating an adequate amount may still seem too scary. They may have muscle injuries or feel sick, yet still feel like a failure if they miss a day of exercise. Often, the issue is not that someone suffering from an eating disorder does not *know* the negative impact of the eating disorder; rather, making the necessary changes and feeling the ensuing discomfort does not feel worth the risk. For this reason, even when it is evident to those around them that their behaviors are harmful and potentially life-threatening, change seems implausible.

Enter group therapy – a place where a group of people can seek help and support together under the supervision of professionals. When one group member can talk about their eating disorder behaviors by expressing a desire for change or acknowledging how the eating disorder has harmed them, it creates the potential for someone else to affirm or support them. This cascade through the group community is powerful; it connects group members through their suffering, experiences, and beliefs that recovery will offer them a fuller life. While sometimes there are issues in the group community, as we thoroughly addressed in Chapter 3, the ability of the group community to instill a shared sense of willingness to feel the discomfort that comes with change trumps the risks.

> "From the very first day, just sharing our fears with each other made it easier to talk and share things with you ladies."
>
> – Former Group Member

## Discussion 4.1 – What's Your Fear?

Group therapy can be a powerful yet uncomfortable place for many. Cultivating a supportive, safe, and meaningful community occurs when members can be forthcoming with one another. Addressing concerns and fears about participating in a group setting is crucial in creating an atmosphere of security and trust. Even a seasoned group participant can have fears that they talk too much, do not talk enough, or could be misunderstood by others. This activity fosters discussion about those worries, which helps create a sense of security and trust and may alleviate the group members' anxieties.

**Begin** by asking each group member to share one fear about being in the group. This fear could be a fear that they will inadvertently say something insensitive to another member and "trigger" them. It may be a fear that they are not sick enough or are too sick for this group. It may be a fear that nobody will talk, and they will not get anything out of the group.

What is one fear you have about being in the group?

**Pause** to allow group members to think of their fear.

**Ask** each person to share their fear aloud. They can include any insights into this fear's origins and underlying meaning.

**Encourage** group members to support each other to identify ways to address the fear (i.e., commit to speaking up if a member feels misunderstood).

Further the discussion by asking:

- What was it like to share your fear?
- What was it like to hear the fears that others shared?
- Has anyone experienced a similar fear (as someone else shared) and found effective strategies to overcome it?
- Has this discussion and specifically talking about these fears helped you feel more at ease towards them? In other words, do you feel differently about this fear now than you did at the start of the group today? If not, are you willing to continue participating in the group despite this fear?

**Address** unresolved fears. If group members still feel anxious or unsettled about their fears, reassure them that ongoing discussions and support will be available in future sessions. Offer to explore individual fears in more depth if indicated (which may include a 1:1 discussion outside the group) or provide additional resources for addressing specific concerns.

### Facilitators' Forum

Suppose one or both group facilitators are part of a group member's treatment team. In that case, that member's fear of being in the group may involve engaging with this clinician in a different setting, "sharing" their provider with others, or even feeling nervous that this clinician may share something about them with the group. We encourage facilitators to review these boundaries with that group member individually before the group to set their mind at ease.

It is up to the group facilitators whether they ask group members not to disclose the names of their treatment team providers. By keeping provider names confidential, group members can avoid potential triggers or emotional distress from knowing their provider has a therapeutic relationship with other group members. This boundary can help maintain psychological safety within the group and prevent disruptions or negative dynamics that could impact the therapeutic process.

## Cohesion

While group cohesion may be described in different ways, there are necessary elements to its definition. In simple terms, it has been described in the literature as a positive bond between group members. For this cohesion to be beneficial, group members and facilitators must have a shared goal of providing support and acceptance.[5]

Each group member should feel that they belong to the group. For group cohesion to occur, members should be able to identify with one another.[6] One simple and effective way to build group cohesion is to have individuals share about themselves. When group members find commonalities in their experience, group cohesion is built. These commonalities are sometimes identified naturally by members themselves or may require the facilitators to help group members recognize their similarities, a skill referred to as linking.[7]

When members feel like they know things about each other, it fosters a sense of connection that becomes the foundation for group cohesion. Group members need not share intimate details about themselves. Even sharing simple information about what type of work someone does, their favorite subject in school, what kind of movies they enjoy watching, or the last vacation they took can foster a sense of intimacy among members.

The stereotype of eating disorders affecting only adolescent white middle-class straight cis-gendered non-disabled girls maintains the shame for those outside these identities. Eating disorders are equal opportunity offenders that affect people of all gender identities, ages, races, ethnicities, body shapes and weights, sexual orientations, socioeconomic statuses, physical abilities, and income levels.[8] In years of co-facilitating our group, we have had newcomers to the group mention feeling embarrassed by the fact they are adults, in some cases with children and leadership positions in their jobs or communities, yet are struggling to take care of themselves in a very fundamental way. Coming to know people they respect and working on their eating disorder recovery can mitigate the shame they feel about having an eating disorder.

We build group cohesion in several ways:

*Ice Breakers:* If you have ever attended a training course or the first day of a program, you are probably familiar with the good ol' icebreaker. This can be a fantastic way to get your group talking, especially a new group that may not feel cohesive (yet!) and may have some difficulty getting started with the conversation. As described earlier, even knowing little things about each other that have nothing to do with the eating disorder can help build a positive bond. Some examples of icebreaker questions include:

- If you could get on a plane today and go anywhere in the world, where would you go and why?
- What was your favorite childhood board game?
- What is a television series you are watching and enjoying now?
- What was the last book you read or podcast you listened to?
- What adjective that starts with the first letter in your first name describes you?

***Taking the Pulse:*** A common way to start our group is with an activity called "Taking the Pulse." This activity consists of an abbreviated check-in, ideally under one minute per person, that allows group members to share how they feel at that moment. As the group builds cohesiveness, members can sense when something is "off" with another member, which can feel disruptive if it is not addressed. For example, suppose someone appears to have low energy because they are not feeling well or are highly anxious because they got into a fender bender on the way to the group. In that case, it is helpful for other group members to know about this.

This activity can replace a check-in, which will be described later, if a long group activity is planned or the group does not have a check-in component.

While we do not always start our group with "taking the pulse," we try to gauge the group ourselves as people enter the room or come on-screen. As you build attunement with your group members, it will be easier to tell when the energy in the physical or virtual room feels different. In these situations, "taking the pulse" before getting started can help members get something off their chest, allowing group members to be sensitive to each other's needs. Examples of these disclosures could include members saying:

- "I'm really excited because I got engaged last night and was so surprised. It was an amazing day and I'm feeling kind of tired because I didn't sleep much last night, but if I look really happy today, that's why. I'll tell the story when it's my turn to check in."
- "I've been sick all week and I'm glad to be in the group today, but it's been rough. I could definitely use the support and I'll check in about it. I may need to step out to use the bathroom at some point."
- "I'm feeling fine today. It's been a pretty normal day. Nothing else to say right now."

***Check-Ins:*** A group check-in refers to a turn-based activity that allows each member to disclose how they are doing. Our group uses it as an opportunity for members to share challenges from their week and any "wins" or "victories," as we refer to them. Members can ask for support from the group if they would like. Sometimes members will share a particular challenge or struggle but will not want support or feedback from the group, which they have the right to communicate.

While group facilitators may feel inclined to provide a professional response to a member's check-in, we encourage them to pause and see if the members talk to each other first. This type of communication is one of the hallmarks that differentiates group therapy from individual therapy. When group facilitators monopolize responses to others and are too verbal in the discussion, the ability of the group to build connections with one another may be hindered.

Whereas "taking the pulse" is a brief opportunity to share specific information, check-in is a longer, more in-depth disclosure. Group facilitators should be aware of the time limitations of the group and how many members are present. For example, suppose you have seven group members in a sixty-minute group. In that case, check-ins will need around five minutes each to allow everyone to share and move on to another activity or discussion. On multiple occasions, our group has prioritized check-ins as the sole focus of our discussions when members delve into deeper, more vulnerable topics. As long as group facilitators ensure ample time for each member to check in and no individual check-in monopolizes the group time, there is nothing wrong with recognizing that what your group needs on that particular day is time to self-disclose and support one another.

While we always come to the group prepared with an activity or discussion to lead after the check-in, often the nature of the conversation and similarities in what members have shared prompts organic and spontaneous discussion. For example, if three members share about body image struggles, it should be apparent to the group facilitators that they need support in this area. In this situation, the check-in provided group facilitators with valuable information about how to best support the group on that day. We hope this book serves as a vital resource in a situation like this by providing a quick body image activity idea or nutrition discussion when needed.

### Integrating New Members

Group facilitators should remember that when a member joins the group, you have one person entering who presumably knows nothing about the other members and everyone else who knows quite a bit about each other. It may feel intimidating to be that new member, stepping into a group that already feels cohesive with established norms. We like to ameliorate this discomfort by spending at least one group doing an activity where group members are encouraged to share something about themselves. Naturally, this deepens what the group already knows about each other and allows the new member to learn something about each pre-existing member. It also shakes up the normal group discussion, making it more approachable and inviting to the new member.

### Activity 4.1 – Eating Disorder Support Group Game Show

This group activity is a favorite among our group. We utilize this Game Show in many ways. Firstly, it is an excellent icebreaker for new members, as it provides an opportunity for everyone to share something about themselves. Secondly, it acts as a conversation starter, helping to stimulate dialogue among group members and keep the conversation flowing.

To set up this activity, facilitators can use index cards to create a game board. Each index card represents a category and a specific point value, such as "Check Out My Skills for 300." Facilitators can write the corresponding question on the back of the card or maintain a separate key with the questions and categories. Arrange the index cards in a grid-like format to resemble a game board, similar to the layout of the TV show "Jeopardy!®" However, the gameplay for this activity is simpler.

During the activity, facilitators will invite group members to take turns choosing a category and point value from the game board. Once a category and point value are selected, the facilitator will read the corresponding question aloud. The questions are designed so that higher point values require more openness and vulnerability from the responses.

To conduct the activity virtually, facilitators can use a virtual game board instead of physical index cards. They can create a digital game board using presentation software, online collaborative tools, or even develop a custom-made game show template. The virtual game board can be shared with the group through screen sharing during the session, allowing participants to make their selections and engage in the activity.

After the group member who selected the questions gives their answer, facilitators may encourage other members to answer that question, fostering rich and meaningful conversation.

It is important to note that completing the entire game board may not be possible within a single group session due to the extensive discussions generated by the activity. If desired, facilitators can continue the activity in subsequent sessions.

## Materials:

- For in-person groups, use index cards, pen, and paper (for facilitators maintaining a list of categories and questions).
- For virtual groups, create a virtual game board to share through screen sharing.

### Categories and Questions

*Check Out My Skills: Exploring Coping Strategies*

100 – What is the main barrier to accessing your coping skills when you have strong urges to use your eating disorder symptoms?

200 – Name three coping skills that have proven helpful for you and describe the situations in which they were particularly effective.

300 – Talk about an "aha" moment where it clicked that using a coping mechanism helped you block using your eating disorder symptom(s). What

challenges do you encounter when attempting to recreate that scenario more frequently?

400 – What is one coping skill you have been interested in trying but have been hesitant to attempt? What factors have contributed to your avoidance of trying it?

500 – Select one new coping mechanism (ideas from the group are welcome) that you will use this week at least once and report back to the group on how it went.

### Relative Revelations: Decoding Family Dynamics

100 – Is there a specific person in your family who has been the most supportive, encouraging, and positive role model during your recovery? If so, how?

200 – How have the family dynamics or the attitudes towards food and body weight or shape within your family influenced your eating disorder and your recovery?

300 – Can you recall a recent incident where a family member or friend made a comment that triggered you? How did you handle the situation, and if given the chance, would you have preferred to handle it differently? If so, how?

400 – What steps have you taken to advocate for your recovery within your family? Measures may include setting boundaries, sharing meals with them, utilizing them for accountability, etc. . . . What approaches have been the most effective in helping your family better understand your journey?

500 – Looking ahead, what specific steps can you take to foster better communication and support from your family in your recovery journey? How can you overcome any barriers or obstacles that have prevented you from taking action in this area?

### The Big Picture: Life Beyond the Eating Disorder

100 – What is one activity or hobby that brings you joy or fulfillment, separate from any thoughts or influences related to your eating disorder?

200 – Reflecting on your eating disorder recovery, describe one moment or experience when you felt a genuine sense of hope and progress. Describe the moment and share how it impacted your motivation and commitment to continue on the path of recovery.

300 – In envisioning a future beyond your eating disorder, what are two aspects of life that you aspire to cultivate and nurture? How do you believe prioritizing your recovery will contribute to realizing these aspirations, and what steps can you take to actively work toward them?

400 – Is there something you have wanted to achieve or accomplish that your eating disorder has prevented you from pursuing? Do you believe it's too late to revisit that aspiration? Explain why or why not.

500 – Imagine that you are at your ninetieth birthday party and someone near and dear to you is getting up to toast you. What do you hope will be said about you and your life? If necessary, what changes would you need to make in your life or how you live to ensure the envisioned remarks become a reality?

### Reflections Explored: Navigating the Realm of Body Image

100 – Despite having "bad body image days," what is one aspect of your body that you genuinely appreciate and can remind yourself of during those moments?

200 – Complete the following sentence: "When I look in the mirror, I'd like to stop feeling ____ and feel ____ instead." What is one action you can take (or may have already taken) to initiate this change and foster a more positive self-perception?

300 – Identify at least two ways you tend to criticize your body. How can you proactively prevent yourself from engaging in these criticisms? Alternatively, is there a healthy way you can respond to that critical inner voice?

400 – Social media impacts our feelings about our bodies and our relationship with food. Have you taken any steps toward having a healthier relationship with social media? If so, what are they? Is there more you can do (and that you are ready and willing to do)?

500 – In recovery, the aim is to shift from being an observer of your body to fully living within it. Your body is no longer an object to be controlled, manipulated, criticized, or changed, but rather the vessel that enables you to navigate life and experience it. Share a memory with the group when you felt liberated from the self-spectator view of your body. What can you do to create more of these embodied experiences?

### Savoring Recovery: Rebuilding a Healthy Connection with Food

100 – Reflecting on the statement, "*Food is fuel. Food is medicine,*" what are the advantages and disadvantages of considering food in these terms for you? How else do you perceive food beyond its functional aspects?

200 – Think of a food that is still feared, avoided, or highly representative of your eating disorder. What steps can you take to normalize your relationship with this specific food and diminish its power over you?

300 – What does a healthy relationship with food look like to you? What are ways you have tried to cultivate this?

400 – Recovery from an eating disorder can be challenging due to the prevalence of media messages promoting diet trends and promising everything from weight loss to enhanced longevity. How has your recovery journey influenced the way you think about and interpret these messages from various media platforms, including social media and news outlets?

500 – Recall a past meal or experience with food that brings back pleasant memories, evoking feelings of fondness, happiness, and contentment. Share this

specific memory with the group, describing the emotions it elicits and the significance it holds for you as you reflect upon it.

### Echoes of Insight: Journeying into My Inner Wisdom

100 – Share a saying, mantra, or words that have resonated with you throughout your eating disorder recovery. It could be a phrase you once heard from someone or something you repeat to yourself daily for inspiration.

200 – Nurturing your well-being requires attentiveness to internal cues. These cues can guide decisions related to eating, resting, and establishing boundaries. What internal cues do you rely on to guide your self-care practices?

300 – List three positive words that describe you as a person unrelated to your appearance. Why do you choose these words?

400 – Recall a recent "sweet spot" moment. Food was going well, body image was okay (maybe even good), or you felt confident that you were living aligned with your values. What lessons or insights can you draw from this experience?

500 – In a culture that often equates appearance, particularly an unrealistic standard of beauty, and following specific eating patterns with personal worth, how can you safeguard your recovery and maintain your sense of value and self-worth?

### Facilitators' Forum

This activity offers facilitators a unique opportunity to assess the topics that resonate with group members and identify any challenges faced by individual members or the entire group. It provides valuable information for thoughtfully planning activities and topics for future groups.

Another benefit of the game show format is that it lends itself to educating. Facilitators can use it as an opportunity to educate participants about relevant topics related to nutrition, mental health, or any other area of focus. Facilitators can include informative questions or discussion points that enhance their knowledge and understanding.

## Fostering Vulnerability

Fostering a sense of trust and safety within the group is pivotal in inspiring vulnerability among its members. However, if individuals perceive a lack of assurance within the group, whether due to breaches in confidentiality or experiences of judgment from a fellow participant or facilitator, the depth of conversation is likely to be compromised, impeding the exploration of sensitive and meaningful topics essential for building authentic connections among the participants.

One effective approach to cultivating trust is for group facilitators to exhibit a willingness to embrace vulnerability. Renowned psychiatrists Sophia Vinogradov and Irvin Yalom noted that group therapists often self-disclose more than individual therapists. This transparency and openness can serve as a genuine demonstration of sincerity and respect.[9] Building trust within relationships necessitates the presence of vulnerability, and it is through trust that participants feel comfortable enough to become vulnerable themselves. Facilitators' self-disclosure should encourage and inspire group members to open up rather than shifting the focus onto the facilitators.

### Activity 4.2 – Discovering the Depths: Introducing Your Inner Struggles

During group conversations and check-ins, group members will gain insights into each other's eating disorder symptoms and challenges. However, some members may find recognizing their unique contributions to the group challenging beyond the expected focus on body image concerns or providing a weekly symptom summary.

This activity offers a creative way to encourage members to share the issues underlying their eating disorders. Doing so allows group members to deepen their understanding of each other and provides group facilitators with valuable topics to explore in future sessions. Examples of such introductions are provided in the Facilitators' Forum.

### Materials:

- For in-person groups, provide paper and writing utensils for group members.
- For virtual groups, members can gather their own writing materials or utilize electronic devices for the activity.

**Introduce** this activity by explaining to participants that they will write an introduction to be shared with the group, focusing on what brought them to the group or their current struggles. Emphasize that this is an opportunity for them to openly express their challenges without referencing weight, shape, size, food, or specific eating disorder symptoms. Encourage them to use metaphors, emotions, or other descriptive elements to convey their experiences. Use the following prompt to guide their introductions:

"Introduce yourself to the group by sharing what brought you to this group or your current struggles. Avoid referring to weight, shape, size, food, or specific eating disorder symptoms. Instead, utilize metaphors, emotions, or other descriptive elements to illuminate the depths of your journey and the obstacles you face."

**Give** approximately five minutes for group members to write. For virtual groups, members may write on paper or type their introduction.

**Allow** members to share their introductions with the group.

**Proceed** with the discussion by asking the following questions. These questions aim to dig deeper into the members' experiences, exploring their reactions, insights, and connections made during the activity.

- Why do you think you were asked to avoid referring to weight, shape, size, food, or specific eating disorder symptoms?
- How did listening to others' introductions make you feel? Additionally, how did it feel to read your introduction aloud?
- Was it challenging to introduce yourself to the group without referencing your eating disorder, body, or food?
- Considering the limitations of the prompt, did you approach your introduction differently than you would have otherwise? If so, how was it different?
- What were some of the underlying themes you noticed in the introductions shared by the group?
- Did this prompt help you identify your eating disorder's underlying functions or purposes?
- Reflecting on your eating disorder through the lens of your introduction, do you believe that your eating disorder serves as an avoidance strategy for these underlying issues? If so, explain.

### Facilitators' Forum

Facilitators may share the following examples of an introduction. These examples serve as a reference, giving members an idea of how to structure and write their own.

Example One: "I don't know my life without my anxiety, the constant ticker in my head, the ever-present flash in my mind pulling my consciousness somewhere else but the here and now. It has affected every relationship in my life causing me to feel misunderstood, isolated, and lonely. No one understands me, and I never feel that I belong. I am afraid to put myself out there, for what if I am rejected? I cannot live the life I want because I am pulled back by the shame I feel and worrying about how others perceive me. Sometimes I feel relief from these worries, but it is at the expense of my physical and mental health. Can I belong here?"

Example Two: "Hello, everyone, I want to share a bit about what brought me to this group. Over the years, I've struggled with feeling like I'm not enough, constantly seeking validation from others. It's as if I've built a fortress around myself, protecting me from the pain of rejection and judgment. This fortress, however, has also kept me isolated and disconnected from my own emotions.

Through this group, I hope to unravel the layers of self-doubt and rediscover my authentic self."

### Activity 4.3 – Group Show and Tell

For some, "show and tell" was an elementary school activity that provided a first experience sharing something about themselves in front of a group. It is a practice of vulnerability, providing an opportunity for self-expression. It can build confidence and connection.

Depending on your group's needs, there are several ways to use this activity, as it naturally serves as a segue to specific topics, including coping skills, identity, and values. The Facilitators' Forum addresses some of the variations of the prompt.

In this instance, members are asked to bring in an object, such as a picture, quote, or anything that holds personal meaning to them that has inspired them in their eating disorder recovery or represents their inspiration. It could be a picture of their child, symbolizing the importance of modeling a healthy relationship with food and body to prevent their child from experiencing the same struggles. Alternatively, it could be a seashell, representing the significance of overcoming body shame that prevented them from enjoying beach time in the past and symbolizing their love for the ocean and the newfound freedom they are discovering.

### Materials:

• For both in-person and virtual groups, each group member will bring one item to share with the group.

**Announce** the activity in the previous group session and ask members to bring something that has inspired them in their eating disorder recovery. Even for a virtual group, announcing the activity beforehand is important. Some participants may not be joining from their homes and may not have their chosen items accessible. Begin by explaining the show-and-tell activity to the group. Let them know that each person will have an opportunity to share an object that has inspired them in their eating disorder recovery. We find it helpful to send a reminder email to ensure all members are prepared and can actively participate.

**Begin** by explaining the show-and-tell activity to the group. Let them know that each person will have an opportunity to share their chosen item and the story behind it, highlighting how it has inspired them during their eating disorder recovery. If desired, each facilitator could model the activity by sharing an object that holds meaning to them in their work as an eating disorder clinician.

> Tell us about what you brought that has inspired you during your eating disorder recovery.

**Invite** each participant to share their object, one at a time. Facilitators might use a round-robin approach, where each person takes a turn sharing, or allow people to volunteer to go one after another. Encourage everyone to ask questions or offer support as appropriate.

**Debrief** the activity as a group after everyone has had a chance to share.

- What insights or reflections did you gain from the stories and symbols shared during the activity?
- Did any of the shared items resonate with you personally? If so, how and why?
- How did this activity contribute to a sense of connection and mutual support within the group?
- Did you discover any new coping skills, values, or aspects of your identity through this activity?

### Facilitators' Forum

Variations of this activity include asking members to share a talent, skill, or passion with the group, such as playing an instrument, reading a favorite poem, or sharing something meaningful to them that has nothing to do with their eating disorder. Suggestions for items include a sentimental photograph, meaningful heirloom, or souvenir from a memorable trip. The rationale for this request is to encourage group members to understand each other and relate on a deeper level beyond their struggles with their eating disorders. This connection helps create community and serves as a powerful reminder that each group member's identity extends beyond their eating disorder.

## Activity 4.4 – Letter to Myself

During this activity, each group member will compose a personal letter addressed to themselves, either to their younger self or present self. Allowing members to address themselves can be a profoundly moving experience as it enables self-exploration, self-disclosure, and self-reflection.

We typically introduce this activity weeks before we share the letters to ensure ample time for introspection and writing. Depending on the group size, it is important to consider that consecutively sharing all the letters may require more than one group session. To maximize this activity over multiple weeks, we recommend designating one or two participants to share their letters per week alongside another separate group activity if indicated.

## Materials:

* For in-person groups, provide paper and writing utensils for group members.
* For virtual groups, members can gather writing materials or utilize electronic devices.

> Write a letter to your younger or present self. In your letter, address the experiences, emotions, or insights relevant to your eating disorder recovery.
> Additionally, please include the following in your letter:
>
> * Reflect on the progress you have made in your recovery so far.
> * Offer words of encouragement, compassion, and support.
> * Share any advice or wisdom you have gained throughout your recovery journey.

**Provide** ample time for group members to write their letters, either during the group session or as assigned homework, as previously mentioned.

**Allow** one person at a time to read their letter aloud to the group.

**Reflect** on each letter by prompting the discussion with questions such as:

* What was the process like for the writer of the letter? Was it hard to get started? Did it come naturally? What emotional experiences were present in the writing? In the reading?
* What was it like to hear this group member's letter? What emotions did you notice feeling?
* How did the content of the letter resonate with your own experiences or recovery?
* Did any particular insights or pieces of advice stand out to you? If so, which ones and why?
* How can we support and validate each other based on the reflections shared in the letters?

### Facilitators' Forum

While the prompt suggests addressing the experiences, emotions, and insights relevant to eating disorder recovery, some participants may feel more comfortable exploring specific themes or aspects of their recovery. Be flexible and open to variations in the letter-writing prompt to accommodate individual preferences. For example, participants may choose to focus on self-acceptance, body image, or specific coping strategies.

## Saying Goodbye

Saying goodbye to group members will occur at different times depending on whether you have a closed group with a time-limited number of sessions or an ongoing group with rolling admission. In a session-limited group, members and group facilitators will say goodbye to each other simultaneously. However, with a rolling admission group, members will inevitably leave at different times. Regardless, creating a ritual to honor these endings can be quite profound.

In life, there is not always an opportunity to recognize endings and for those endings to be deliberate and positive. They may be associated with a painful loss, abandonment, rejection, and separation. In an ongoing group, participants are asked to tell the group facilitators when they would like to leave the group. Not only is this beneficial as it allows the departing member to say goodbye to the group, but it also promotes attachment security. When participants know that group members do not simply show up in one group and are gone the next without notice, they may feel more comfortable investing in the group, being vulnerable, and building trust. Termination rituals give members different, and possibly corrective, emotional experiences they can take from the group into their lives.

Taking time to honor members' contributions to the group acknowledges their value and how they left a mark on the community. In the following rituals, the group member(s) leaving will have a chance to hear positive feedback and supportive words. Allowing group members to speak directly to the participant(s) leaving can be a powerful and meaningful experience they will always remember.

## Activity 4.5 – Hope and Gratitude

This activity is designed to celebrate and honor a departing group member. It allows participants to express their hope and gratitude to this member, creating a lasting reminder of their presence within the group. As part of the activity, the departing group member is asked to offer a hope and gratitude to themself, reminding them of their worth and the positive impact they have had on the group.

For an in-person group, this is an opportunity to give members something tangible they can take with them. It becomes a physical reminder of the group. It could be a card passed around during the last session where members and facilitators identify hopes and gratitude directly to the member leaving. Another option would be to have a member act as a scribe for the group and write down these hopes and gratitude on a single piece of paper as members share them.

For virtual groups, there may not be a tangible component to this activity. Instead, group members may verbally share their hope and gratitude for the exiting member. Members can also email their hope and gratitude for the departing member and email them to a facilitator who can compile them. If a group member is absent for this ritual, it is important to get their hope and gratitude ahead of time so the facilitator can read it in their absence.

## Materials:

• For in-person groups, use paper and colored markers if desired.

> As we mark [name]'s departure from our group, let's each share words of hope for them as well as gratitude.

**Ask** each group member to take a minute and think about their hope and gratitude for the departing group member.

**Facilitate** the sharing process, going around the group and allowing each participant and the facilitators to express their hope and gratitude.

**Conclude** the activity by asking the departing group member to grant *themselves* hope and gratitude. Although this may feel uncomfortable for them, this exercise allows group members to practice self-compassion, a skill we will discuss more in Chapter 5.

### Facilitators' Forum

An example of a hope and appreciation from a group member may sound like this:

"My hope for [departing member] is that they will have the courage to tell their partner more about their eating disorder. It has been inspiring to hear you feel increasingly ready to do this and I believe you can. My gratitude for you is how attentive you are during group. I feel like you always listened deeply to everyone; because of this, I felt how important this community was to you. I will really miss you."

An example of a group member's hope and gratitude for themselves may sound like this:

"My hope for myself is that I will find the peace with my body that I know is possible. This group has allowed me to hear the voices of others who are working on accepting their bodies and I have felt less alone. My gratitude for myself is that I came to the group each week. Sometimes it was hard to get here and I felt like there were other things I needed to do, but I'm grateful that I prioritized this experience."

## Activity 4.6 – Goodbye Letters

This activity is intended for session-limited groups with a predetermined end date. It is a simple yet powerful activity where members are encouraged to write a letter to the group. In this letter, they can express what the group experience has meant to them and what they have gained from being a part of the group.

Be prepared for emotions to run high during this activity, as it often evokes heartfelt responses. In groups that have developed a strong sense of community and cohesion, the impact of these letters can be particularly moving.

Facilitators can assign this as homework. For in-person or virtual groups, members can bring their completed letters to the final group. Alternatively, facilitators can provide dedicated time during the group for members to write their letters.

This activity is an opportunity for group members to reflect on their personal growth, express gratitude for the support received, and acknowledge the connections formed within the group. It can be a powerful closing ritual that honors the shared journey and the transformative impact of the group experience.

### Materials:

• For in-person groups, provide paper and writing utensils for group members.
• For virtual groups, members can gather their own writing materials or utilize electronic devices for the activity.

Whether assigning the letter as homework or introducing it in a group session, provide the following prompt:

> Write a goodbye letter to the group. Consider including what you have learned from the group, what you have appreciated about the group and group members, and what you will remember most about this experience.

**Proceed** around the room and allow group members to share their letters aloud.

**Reflect and summarize** the key points or themes that emerged after all members have shared. This process is valuable as it validates their experiences and assists participants in recognizing the commonalities and connections within the group.

**Conclude** the activity by expressing gratitude for the group and its members. Facilitators can take this opportunity to share their reflections, underscoring the significant progress and growth witnessed within the group. Emphasize the collective achievements and positive dynamics that have emerged throughout the sessions. Acknowledging and celebrating these accomplishments further reinforces the sense of unity, resilience, and support cultivated within the group.

*Facilitators' Forum*

If facilitators decide to recognize individuals' progress, it is essential to do so for all participants, ensuring equal acknowledgment and validation of each person's unique journey. Recognizing and celebrating each participant's progress can profoundly impact their self-esteem. It fosters a supportive and validating environment where everyone's growth is honored and valued.

Facilitators need to be mindful of any potential biases or unintentional favoritism that may arise. By consciously ensuring that every participant receives equal recognition and validation, facilitators uphold fairness and encourage a safe and supportive space for all members.

## Activity 4.7 – Box of Trinkets

This activity provides a creative way to honor a departing member. By harnessing the power of metaphors, group members come together to bestow symbolic gifts to the transitioning member. By the end of the group, a cherished "box of trinkets" will be created, symbolizing the collective support within the group.

In addition to the gifts from others, the departing member is invited to give themselves a symbolic gift. They are encouraged to reflect on their personal growth, achievements, and strengths experienced throughout their time in the group. This self-gift becomes a meaningful reminder of their progress and group experience.

At the end of the activity, the compiled symbolic gifts can be presented to the departing member. This gesture is a tangible representation of the group's support, gratitude, and appreciation for the individual. It captures the group's shared experiences, bonds, and heartfelt wishes, leaving a lasting impression and fostering a sense of belonging and connection even after their departure.

In in-person groups, participants can write their symbolic gifts on paper or note cards during the session. These cards can be passed around, allowing everyone to contribute their thoughts. Alternatively, for virtual or in-person groups, facilitators can suggest that participants send their written gifts before the session. Once gathered, facilitators can create a visually appealing document that combines all the symbolic gifts electronically or in print. This memento symbolizes the group's unity and can inspire and motivate the departing member as they move forward.

## Materials:

- For in-person groups, provide paper or note cards with markers or other coloring utensils.
- For virtual groups, facilitators can compile an electronic card (see activity introduction).

**Begin** this termination ritual by acknowledging that it is the final group session for the departing member. Explain the process, stating that each participant will take turns presenting their symbolic gift and inviting the departing member to give themselves a symbolic gift.

> Today we will mark [name]'s departure from our group by each sharing a symbolic gift for them.

**Proceed** around the room (or virtual room), allowing each member a chance to give their gift.

Some examples are:

- "I want to give you headphones that repeatedly play words of encouragement."
- "I want to give you a baseball bat so that you can smash the scale in your bathroom!"

**Invite** the departing member to reflect on the gifts they have received. Encourage them to express their emotions, insights, and gratitude.

**Facilitate** a discussion highlighting common themes or patterns in the symbolic gifts, fostering a sense of connection and validation.

### Facilitators' Forum

Facilitators can offer ideas or guiding questions to help participants generate meaningful and appropriate symbolic gifts for the departing member. These prompts serve to focus their thinking and ensure that the gifts align with the purpose of the activity, which is to honor and celebrate the individual leaving the group.

For example, you can offer prompts such as:

- "Consider a moment or experience shared with the departing member that significantly impacted you. What symbolic gift could represent that moment?"
- "Reflect on the growth and progress the departing member has made during their time in the group. What symbol or object could embody that transformation?"
- "Think about something that you hope for the departing group member. What is a symbolic gift that could represent that hope?"

## Notes

1 Wanlass, Janine, J. Kelly Moreno, and Hannah M. Thomson. 2005. "Group Therapy for Eating Disorders: A Retrospective Case Study." *The Journal for Specialists in Group Work* 30 (1): 47–66. https://doi.org/10.1080/01933920590908697.

2  Grenon, Renee, Dominique Schwartze, Nicole Hammond, Iryna Ivanova, Nancy Mcquaid, Genevieve Proulx, and Giorgio A. Tasca. 2017. "Group Psychotherapy for Eating Disorders: A Meta-Analysis." *International Journal of Eating Disorders* 50 (9): 997–1013. https://doi.org/10.1002/eat.22744.
3  Horvath, Adam O. 2001. "The Alliance." *Psychotherapy: Theory, Research, Practice, Training* 38 (4): 365–372. https://doi.org/10.1037/0033-3204.38.4.365.
4  Christensen, Anne Bryde, Signe Wahrén, Nina Reinholt, Stig Poulsen, Morten Hvenegaard, Erik Simonsen, and Sidse Arnfred. 2021. " 'Despite the Differences, We Were All the Same'. Group Cohesion in Diagnosis-Specific and Transdiagnostic CBT Groups for Anxiety and Depression: A Qualitative Study." *International Journal of Environmental Research and Public Health* 18 (10): 5324. https://doi.org/10.3390/ijerph18105324.
5  Harpine, Elaine Clanton. 2010. "Group Cohesion: The Therapeutic Factor in Groups." *Group-Centered Prevention Programs for At-Risk Students*: 117–140. https://doi.org/10.1007/978-1-4419-7248-4_9.
6  Christensen et al., "Despite the Differences," 2021.
7  Novotney, Amy. 2019. "Keys to Great Group Therapy." *Monitor on Psychology* 50 (4). www.apa.org/monitor/2019/04/group-therapy.
8  Schaumberg, Katherine, Elisabeth Welch, Lauren Breithaupt, Christopher Hübel, Jessica H. Baker, Melissa A. Munn-Chernoff, Zeynep Yilmaz, et al. 2017. "The Science behind the Academy for Eating Disorders' Nine Truths about Eating Disorders." *European Eating Disorders Review* 25 (6): 432–450. https://doi.org/10.1002/erv.2553.
9  Vinogradov, Sophia, and Irvin D. Yalom. 1990. "Self-Disclosure in Group Psychotherapy." In *Self-Disclosure in the Therapeutic Relationship*, edited by George Stricker and Martin Fisher, 191–204. New York: Springer. https://doi.org/10.1007/978-1-4899-3582-3_13.

# Chapter 5

# Taking Care of Myself Without the Eating Disorder

## Developing Self-Care Practices

Learning to care for oneself without relying on disordered thoughts and behaviors is vital to recovering from an eating disorder. This chapter explores the interplay between eating disorders and the underlying needs they strive to fulfill, such as control, comfort, and emotional numbing.

Practical tools and strategies to address these needs are introduced, empowering group members to break free from harmful eating disorder behaviors. This exploration provides an understanding of how eating disorders have functioned as coping mechanisms, aiming to alleviate the burden of shame. It underscores the importance of nurturing and adopting appropriate self-care habits as an essential component of sustainable recovery. Sample group activities and discussion guides are provided.

This chapter integrates a range of therapeutic approaches to provide comprehensive support for group members. The evidence-based techniques and strategies address the multidimensional aspects of eating disorders, encompassing the emotional, cognitive, and behavioral domains.

Cognitive-Behavioral Therapy (CBT) techniques are utilized to challenge and modify unhelpful thoughts and behaviors associated with the eating disorder. Mindfulness-based practices are incorporated to cultivate present-moment awareness, acceptance, and self-compassion. Dialectical Behavior Therapy (DBT) principles are applied to enhance emotional regulation and interpersonal effectiveness. Psychoeducation provides knowledge and understanding of eating disorders, their impact, and the recovery process.

The chapter is also informed by Compassion-Focused Therapy (CFT), which aims to foster self-compassion and reduce self-criticism. Additionally, principles from Positive Psychology are integrated to promote well-being, resilience, and the cultivation of strengths. The therapeutic approach also draws insights from Internal Family Systems (IFS) and incorporates mindfulness techniques to facilitate self-awareness and inner healing.

DOI: 10.4324/9781003430964-8

## Reclaiming Self-Care Without the Eating Disorder

The eating disorder is, in essence, a fraudulent and harmful form of self-care that individuals with eating disorders learn to rely on. It often develops quite innocently. For some, it may have been an effort to become "healthier" that snowballed and became the antithesis of health.

On the surface, a person's eating disorder may appear to be about food and weight. For many, food and weight become a way to cope with distressing emotions, such as anxiety or depression. Food restriction, binge eating, or purging by self-induced vomiting or exercise can provide temporary control and comfort, numbing or alleviating emotional pain. Although the roots of eating disorders are multifaceted and complex, the emergence of these behaviors is intricately connected to a person's desire to ameliorate the discomfort and thus care for themselves. As a result of the enduring nature of their eating disorder symptoms, it is common for those grappling with eating disorders to feel at a loss, uncertain about how to engage in self-care that does not involve their disordered behaviors.

Introducing members to the idea that their eating disorder has served them in some way can be eye-opening and shame-abating. It feels easy to keep falling back on the same behaviors that make someone feel secure and cared for, even if they are harmful. Abandoning these behaviors can feel deeply unsettling, so implementing helpful, nurturing, and appropriate self-care habits (in their absence) is necessary. Looking at the persistence of eating disorders through this lens, one can understand how they can last for years, even decades, of a person's life.

## Activity 5.1 – Self-Care Defined

Diet culture, consumerism, and eating disorders have co-opted self-care by promoting a distorted view of the body that prioritizes external appearance over genuine well-being. The rise of the internet and social media have allowed these harmful ideologies to spread and become more pervasive, perpetuating the idea that self-care encompasses achieving a certain body type, following a strict diet, or buying products that promise to improve one's appearance.

This commodification of self-care reinforces the notion that worth is tied to physical appearance and promotes the idea that bodies must constantly be managed and improved upon. However, expanding the definition of self-care beyond materialistic indulgences is essential to help individuals develop pragmatic, healthy self-care practices.

Facilitators can assist group members in conceptualizing a more expansive definition of self-care that prioritizes emotional and physical health. Self-care includes setting healthy boundaries, tending to basic physical and emotional needs, and listening to their bodies. This shift in mindset can help group members create personalized self-care routines that are sustainable, meaningful, and aligned with their values.

## Materials:

- For in-person groups, use a whiteboard or oversized piece of paper and a writing utensil.
- For virtual groups, facilitators will use a virtual whiteboard or chat box.

**Introduce** the topic by sharing some of the previous education on the connection between self-care and recovery. Encourage group members to consider a more expansive definition of self-care than consumerism or pampering.

Ask the prompt:

> What comes to mind when you hear the phrase "self-care?" How would you define it?

**Write** these definitions on a whiteboard or flip chart (or for virtual groups on a virtual whiteboard or chat box).

**Explain** that while there have been many definitions for the concept of self-care proposed over time, there is not one definitive definition. The following criteria will inform the understanding of self-care for this discussion. For in-person groups, it may be helpful for facilitators to write these down for all group members to see. For virtual groups, facilitators can adapt this approach by utilizing the chat box or a virtual whiteboard feature.

- Self-care refers to the "ability to refill and refuel oneself in healthy ways."[1]
- Self-care practices may be defined as "engagement in behaviors that maintain and promote physical and emotional well-being and may include factors such as sleep, exercise, use of social support, emotion regulation strategies, and mindfulness practice."[2]
- Self-care is the "multidimensional, multifaceted process of purposeful engagement in strategies that promote healthy functioning and enhance well-being."[3]

**Reflect** on how the diet industry, fitness industry, consumerism, and members' eating disorders have co-opted self-care and how this has impacted their self-care practices.

**Identify** self-care practices that prioritize emotional and physical health and are not informed by diet culture or their eating disorders. Examples may include meditation, walking in nature, spending time with loved ones, or journaling.

### Facilitators' Forum

Ask group members to commit to trying one different form of self-care this week at least one time. Group members may share their experiences with the group at the start of the following session.

## The Function of the Eating Disorder

The eating disorder helps many cope with difficult emotions or situations, such as anxiety, depression, trauma, or low self-esteem. It may have provided a sense of control, competence, or a way to numb or distract from painful feelings.

Fear, shame, guilt, and a sense of loss may arise when considering recovery. It can feel like losing a trusted companion, security blanket, or even a part of oneself. Understanding and acknowledging the function of the eating disorder can help group members let go of their attachment to it and find alternative ways to meet their needs.

## Activity 5.2: Exploring the Function of My Eating Disorder

This activity aims to facilitate a deeper understanding of how the eating disorder serves as a coping mechanism and to develop alternative coping strategies that are healthier and feel effective. By gaining insight into their triggers, members can build self-compassion, decreasing shame and increasing awareness of genuine needs and desires.

The eating disorder once served as a resourceful coping mechanism driven by an attempt to address underlying emotional, physical, or relational needs. It is crucial for facilitators to emphasize that the group members' needs are not the problem. Rather, the problem lies in the extreme measures taken to fulfill those needs.

## Materials:

- Worksheet "Exploring the Function of My Eating Disorder" (Appendix 5A)
- For in-person groups, provide paper and writing utensils for group members.
- For virtual groups, members can gather their own writing materials or utilize electronic devices for the activity.

**Invite** group members to take some time to reflect on what purposes their eating disorder has served in their life and how it currently serves them. Examples may include coping with difficult emotions, gaining a sense of control, seeking validation, or eliciting attention from others.

**Use** the worksheet "Exploring the Function of My Eating Disorder" (Appendix 5A) to guide discussion around this topic.

> What functions do your eating disorder serve?

**Further** the conversation to discern functions that can be met in other ways (without the use of the eating disorder) and needs that in actuality are not necessary at all when a healthier sense of self is developed. For example, gaining a sense of control over life could be addressed in other ways, such as keeping a more efficient schedule, making a daily to-do list, and tackling some avoided tasks. However, gaining feelings of competence or superiority over others may become less relevant or necessary as someone's sense of self strengthens in their recovery.

**Focus on** validating group members' needs and showing themselves and each other compassion as they work on developing alternative self-care strategies that can provide similar benefits without the harmful consequences of their eating disorders. Developing these new strategies may involve exploring and identifying unhealthy narratives that maintain their eating disorders, replacing them with expansive and values-driven ones, and engaging in self-care practices that promote healing.

### Facilitators' Forum

One way to help group members identify the functions of their eating disorders is to ask them to imagine committing to never using any eating disorder symptoms again. This question may lead to anxiety, which can be explored by asking, *What do you fear you may have to feel? What do you fear would happen?*

## Activity 5.3: Adventures in Self-Care

People sometimes get into a rut of reverting to the same self-care practices over and over, even if they no longer have a strong interest in the activity or it has grown dull with time. Often something is getting in the way of pursuing unexplored interests or ideas to try something new. This activity aims to encourage group members to broaden their thinking around self-care practices and identify potential barriers to trying new forms of self-care. In doing so, members continue to expand their self-care repertoire and hopefully feel renewed enthusiasm in their recovery.

While the understanding that eating disorder behaviors have no place in recovery may seem obvious, it holds a deeper significance. It signifies the vital need to develop new coping skills as a fundamental aspect of the healing process. These coping skills encompass body-related activities, such as solving puzzles or enjoying the outdoors, along with intentional actions that shape our environment and routines to cultivate a sense of self-care, like prioritizing relaxation, listening to one's body, responding appropriately to its signals, and establishing healthy boundaries.

## Materials:

- Worksheet "Adventures in Self-Care" (Appendix 5B)
- For in-person groups, provide paper and writing utensils for group members.
- For virtual groups, members can gather their own writing materials or utilize electronic devices for the activity.

**Introduce** the topic of self-care and its importance in eating disorder recovery.

**Use** "Adventures in Self-Care" (Appendix 5B), which asks participants to identify activities they are currently comfortable practicing, activities they want to try but have not yet, and activities they want to try but are afraid of or avoid.

> What self-care activities am I comfortable practicing?
> What activities do I want to try but have not yet?
> What activities do I want to try but am afraid of or am avoiding?

**Ask** participants to share their lists with the group and encourage discussion around the following questions:

- What are the benefits of practicing self-care in eating disorder recovery?
- What are some common barriers to practicing self-care, and how can they be addressed?
- How can self-care practices be integrated into daily life and routine?
- What keeps you from trying some of the activities in the third column? Do you believe you will not be "good" at it, will not be accepted into a group (if it is a group activity), or is it not the right use of your time?

**Create**, as a group, a collective list of self-care activities and strategies that group members can draw from in their recovery.

**Assign** homework, if desired, by asking participants to choose one self-care activity from their list that they are comfortable practicing and one that they want to try but have yet to. Encourage them to plan to incorporate these practices into their daily or weekly routine, whichever is applicable, and reflect on any challenges or successes.

**Remind** participants to approach self-care with self-compassion and openness to experimentation rather than rigid expectations or pressures.

### Facilitators' Forum

Forms of self-care that may arise during this activity include exercise and cooking. Both of these activities have the potential to fulfill one's self-care needs independently, separate from any influence from the eating disorder. However, it is essential to recognize that there can be a subtle distinction between engaging in these activities for genuine self-care and having exercise become intertwined with eating disorder behaviors. It is important to remind the group that when exercise, cooking, or other physically demanding activities are done with the intention of or focus on changing the size or shape of one's body, they cease to be acts of self-care.

## Self-Compassion and Self-Care

Research indicates that people with eating disorders or concerns related to their eating habits, body image, and weight tend to experience high levels of self-criticism, self-directed hostility, and shame.[4] In addition, these individuals may encounter difficulties in developing and expressing emotions associated with self-soothing and building supportive relationships with others.[5] All of these factors contribute to feelings of isolation and disconnection.

Enter self-compassion. Research shows that self-compassion can help reduce self-criticism and increase feelings of self-worth, promoting a sense of inner peace, kindness, social connectedness, and emotion regulation.[6] Additionally, individuals who regularly engage in self-compassion may develop a greater capacity for self-soothing during times of stress.[7]

Practicing self-compassion is associated with improved body image and reduced disordered eating.[8] Also, self-compassion is positively associated with body appreciation, body acceptance, and a healthy relationship with food.[9]

## Activity 5.4: Dear Me, I'm Here for You

Recovery is a process and with that can come treatment fatigue. Taking time to acknowledge the progress that group members have made and having them offer themselves words of encouragement can combat that fatigue and help retain motivation and hope in recovery. Engaging in self-reflection allows group members to cultivate self-compassion, self-validation, and self-care.

In this letter-writing activity, group members can explore and cultivate a greater sense of compassion toward themselves. By intentionally expressing kind and encouraging words in their letters, participants can actively contribute to rewiring their brains toward a more positive, optimistic, and resilient mindset. This process allows the exploration of new perspectives, the reinforcement of empowering beliefs, and the fostering of a more confident and compassionate self-image.

### Materials:

- For in-person groups, provide paper and writing utensils for group members.
- For virtual groups, members can gather their own writing materials or utilize electronic devices for the activity.

**Invite** participants to take a few moments to reflect on their eating disorder recovery thus far. Encourage them to consider their strengths, accomplishments, and the challenges they have faced.

**Ask** participants to write a letter of encouragement to themselves. The letter can be written in whatever format feels most comfortable, but it should include specific words of affirmation, kindness, and support. Encourage participants to be gentle with themselves and avoid negative self-talk. They should imagine that they are speaking to a friend who is going through a difficult time. What words of encouragement or advice would they give to them? Write down that encouragement and advice as if they are giving it to themselves.

- To highlight the theme of self-compassion and self-validation, facilitators may ask group members to consider questions such as: *What have been some of the biggest challenges you've faced in your eating disorder recovery? What are some things you are proud of yourself for accomplishing? What are some things you are grateful for about yourself and your treatment/recovery efforts thus far? What are some ways you can show yourself kindness and support as you continue on this path of recovery? How can you celebrate your progress and accomplishments, no matter how small they may seem?*

> Using words of affirmation, kindness, and support, write a letter of encouragement to yourself.

**Allow** time for group members to write their letters and then invite them to share their letters or excerpts from their letters if they are not comfortable sharing them in their entirety.

**Reflect** on the activity and any insights group members gained from writing the letter and hearing other members' letters. To facilitate discussion, ask questions such as:

- What was the process of writing your letter like for you?
- Did any insights or new information emerge as you wrote your letter?
- Were there any challenges or resistance you experienced during the process? How did you overcome them?
- How did you feel reading your letter aloud to the group? How did it feel to hear others' letters? Did anything resonate with you?
- How can you incorporate the messages of encouragement and support from your letter into your daily life and recovery?

### Facilitators' Forum

Encourage group members to consider sending their letter to themselves by mail or keeping it in an easily accessible place, such as a journal or a special box. This provides an opportunity for group members to have a tangible reminder of their self-compassion, support, and encouragement during challenging times.

## Activity 5.5: Nurturing Self-Care in Eating Disorder Recovery

A regular, fulfilling self-care practice is crucial for all people, especially those who struggle with eating disorders due to the disconnect they may feel from their bodies and emotions. This lack of attunement can obscure one's sense of what they truly need in a given moment and make certain self-care categories difficult to practice.

This activity aims to assist group members in identifying various forms of self-care within three categories. Participants are encouraged to reflect on the emotions associated with these self-care practices and evaluate whether they allocate sufficient time for them. Discussion questions are provided to deepen the conversation.

## Materials:

- Worksheet "Nurturing Self-Care in Eating Disorder Recovery" (Appendix 5C)
- For in-person groups, provide paper and writing utensils for group members.
- For virtual groups, members can gather their own writing materials or utilize electronic devices for the activity.

**Begin** by educating the group members about the significance of self-care in the recovery process. Explain that self-care involves actively engaging in practices that promote physical, emotional, and spiritual well-being.

**Use** the worksheet "Nurturing Self-Care in Eating Disorder Recovery" (Appendix 5C) and allow group members about five to ten minutes to complete it.

> How do you engage in self-care to promote your physical, emotional, and spiritual needs?

**Review** the worksheet as a group and encourage members to share their answers aloud.

**Further** the discussion on self-care by asking:

- How do you decide which category of self-care to use at any given moment? What cues or feelings do you notice that might sway you toward one category in particular?
- Is there ever a time when self-care does not feel good to you (e.g., feeling selfish with time or difficulty prioritizing it over other commitments)? If so, what are the barriers to feeling good while engaging in self-care and how might you address them?
- Assess your current commitment to self-care. Do you allocate enough time to practices that are important to you? If not, reflect on the reasons behind this. If you do, what strategies or routines have been effective for you?

### Facilitators' Forum

Facilitators should note that some members may not have three answers for each self-care category. In fact, some may not have any answers. If so, facilitators should encourage group members to be compassionate toward themselves and add ideas to their lists as they hear about self-care practices that may interest them during the discussion.

## Activity 5.6: Unpacking Vacation

A vacation represents a reprieve from life's typical stressors. Taking time off from work, staying in a place away from home, and getting to experience fun excursions or relaxation can elicit a sense of contentment and even calm. Going a layer deeper and having our needs met in different ways can often highlight how we care for ourselves in the first place. Did we enjoy walking to the local coffee shop each morning to pick up a piping hot cup of coffee? How about relaxing by playing a board game with others in the evening instead of doing chores or other mundane tasks?

When people return to their daily lives, does all of the excitement, mystery, or luxury of vacation have to dissolve? This activity will help members identify ways they care for themselves in a setting where self-care is more normalized, even expected, and prompt them to consider whether and how these things can be incorporated into their everyday lives. This activity is rooted in the principles of self-care and self-compassion.

### Materials:

- Worksheet "Unpacking Vacation" (Appendix 5D)
- For in-person groups, provide paper and writing utensils for group members.
- For virtual groups, members can gather their own writing materials or utilize electronic devices for the activity.

**Guide** members to identify an enjoyable vacation that they have taken. It may not necessarily be their most recent one.

**Use** "Unpacking Vacation" (Appendix 5D) and ask group members to write down some habits, actions, or intentions from the vacation that made them feel cared for or simply feel good. If needed, provide examples such as sitting on the beach for a few quiet minutes in the morning, reading before bed, or conversing with friends or family.

> **What habits, actions, or intentions from a past vacation made you feel cared for or generally feel good?**

The second column of the worksheet is a place to gather words describing this self-care action's overarching theme. For example, if a member puts reading before bed as their action, some words that pertain to this may be *slow down, drift,* and *peace.*

**Further** the activity by asking members:

- If caring for yourself required implementing more of the second column words into your life, how might you accomplish that?
- What feels doable? What feels out of reach?
- Do you tell yourself anything that keeps you from trying any of the actions you can think of?
- Could you do what you did on vacation or is there a different thing you could do to feel this way more often?

**Encourage** group members to think about what they could commit to trying between now and the next group session. Focus on small commitments that seem achievable at this moment.

*Facilitators' Forum*

It is expected that members will have recollections that involve food, yet it is normal for them to feel conflicted about the role that food or their eating disorder may have played in those experiences. The dietitian can deepen the conversation by highlighting if and how food enhances the experience or memory. The member may be able to think about the food or experience differently now than they were able to at the time. The dietitian can probe into how their relationship with food has changed since then. How does this change inform the choices they make around food today? This can then be a segue into a broader discussion about finding pleasure and joy in food again, as Registered Dietitians Evelyn Tribole and Elyse Resch discuss in their well-known book, *Intuitive Eating: A Revolutionary Anti-Diet Approach.*[10]

## Activity 5.7: Pocket-Sized Positivity

In this activity, group members will work together to brainstorm a list of essential tools, principles, or strategies that they consider critical to their eating disorder recovery. This list might include positive, motivating statements or reference valuable coping skills, such as self-compassion and mindfulness. Facilitators will transform this list into compact credit card-sized notes, ensuring each group member has a tangible reminder of their shared wisdom. To provide a glimpse of the final product, Image 5.1 showcases a sample card created by a past group.

Facilitators can compile this list and share it electronically to ensure that group members who participate virtually, don't carry wallets, or prefer digital reminders can still access their essential tools and strategies. By having physical or digital reminders of these tools, group members can be frequently reminded of the support and encouragement provided by the group, even when they are not physically present. This collaboratively created list fosters community and connection among the members, reinforcing the understanding that recovery is not a solitary journey. By promoting self-efficacy and empowerment in the context of a supportive group environment, this activity can help participants feel more confident and capable in their ability to navigate the challenges of eating disorder recovery.

## Materials:

- Group facilitators will need writing materials or to utilize electronic devices to make note of suggestions for the card.
- If creating a physical card for each group member, facilitators will need paper, a printer, and laminator if desired. If creating a digital card, an electronic device is required.

**Explain** the activity in its entirety so that members understand the goal of creating a tangible or digital card for themselves.

**Gather** affirmations, mantras, or other positive pieces of wisdom. Facilitators may decide that each group member will come up with one, or the group could brainstorm collectively. The facilitators can transcribe the ideas. There is no right or wrong way to do this.

What affirmations, mantras, or other positive pieces of wisdom or coping skills have resonated with you in recovery?

**Decide** how many and which statements will go on the card.

(Outside the group, facilitators should create either a tangible or digital card that includes the statements the group came up with. If facilitators are making a card to give to group members, we recommend laminating them to distribute at the following group session.

**Encourage** group members to use the cards as a means of support and inspiration when they need positive motivation in recovery.

### Facilitators' Forum

This activity can be fitting for a fixed-session group as they near the end of the cycle. Asking group members what key messages they will take away from their group experience or what moments were most meaningful to them are examples of questions to ask to identify good content for the card. If this activity is done during the last group of the cycle, facilitators could mail a physical card to each group member or email a virtual card after the last session.

**Have a sense of humor-** An asset to help me see the big picture and put things into perspective.
**Follow a schedule -** For daily schedule and meals, and allow for flexibility to go with the flow when appropriate.
**Make self-care a priority-** Listen to my body and make my needs a priority.
**Be your own best mom-** Practice self-compassion and use a curious, non-judgemental stance to understand the functions of my ED urges.
**Communicate honestly-** Be open with myself and others regarding ED urges and behavior.
**Challenge perfectionism-** Be okay with just being okay and sit with feelings.
**Set boundaries-** Foster healthy relationships by setting boundaries regarding food and exercise talk, social media, and ED behaviors. Curate life and social media to be as free of diet culture as possible.
**Be patient-** Know that recovery takes a long time, but I am always progressing on my journey.
**Know my anchors-** Understand my values and what is most important to me. Let these things help me to see what is most important in my life even when I am struggling.
**Zoom out-** Don't lose sight of the "big picture." Not everything is *that* important.

*Figure 5.1* Sample "pocket-sized positivity card" from a past group.

## Meditation Practice for Self-Care

Using guided meditation in eating disorder recovery has benefits such as decreasing stress and anxiety levels and improving body image and one's relationship with their body. These benefits are achieved through present-moment awareness, cultivating self-compassion, detaching from unhelpful thoughts, and building a sense of connection between the mind and body.

The first step in this meditation practice involves finding a comfortable seated position and taking deep breaths in and out. This technique is commonly used in mindfulness-based approaches and is found to be effective in treating eating disorders.[11] By focusing on the present moment, group members can develop a sense of grounding and calmness, which can help alleviate stress and anxiety and promote greater self-awareness and self-compassion.

Visualizing the inner child and using affirmations like "You can trust me to take care of you" and "I am here to be compassionate with you" are consistent with the principles of IFS. IFS conceptualizes the human psyche as comprising multiple subpersonalities, each with its own unique characteristics and needs. Using this lens, the child part of an individual often holds internalized core beliefs that cause emotional pain, which may be driving eating disorder behaviors in an attempt to protect that child from further harm.

By approaching this part with compassion and curiosity, group members are more likely to understand and address underlying emotional pain, develop greater empathy and emotional regulation, and are less likely to turn to harmful coping mechanisms, such as disordered eating.

Finally, the visualization of embracing the inner child with love and care draws upon principles from CFT, which emphasizes the importance of cultivating self-compassion and kindness toward oneself. Research has shown that individuals who exhibit higher levels of self-compassion tend to experience a greater sense of acceptance and appreciation for their bodies while experiencing less preoccupation with their bodies, less overall dissatisfaction with the body, and fewer concerns related to food and body.[12]

## Activity 5.8 – Calming Care Meditation

Meditation has numerous benefits for decreasing stress and anxieties related to eating disorders. However, initiating a meditation practice can be challenging for individuals who struggle with quieting their mind or have concerns about it being boring. Utilizing guided meditation can help address these concerns by providing a structured framework with clear instructions, making it more accessible for beginners to engage in the practice and maintain focus. The guided format supports group members in staying present and actively participating in the meditation, enhancing their ability to experience the benefits of the practice.

### Facilitator Script

Start by finding a comfortable position in a chair with your back straight and your hands resting on your lap. Take a deep breath in, and slowly exhale.

As you sit here, I want you to bring to mind an image of yourself when you were a child. See yourself playing, laughing, and enjoying life without worries or fears.

But also recognize that this child may have felt something was wrong with them, felt inadequate, or may have felt their body was a problem or potentially could be. Allow this image to become as vivid as possible in your mind.

Now, I want you to visualize yourself sitting here with the group in the present moment. Imagine yourself surrounded by the supportive and caring individuals here with you today.

As you sit here, take a moment to connect with your inner child. See them standing before you, looking up at you with trusting eyes.

As you look at this child part of yourself, I want you to repeat the following affirmations to them:

"You can trust me to take care of you."
"I validate your feelings and experiences."
"I am here to be compassionate with you."
"I set you free to be playful and enjoy life."

Repeat these affirmations to your inner child a few times, allowing them to sink in and resonate within you both.

Now, I want you to visualize yourself embracing your inner child, holding them close in a loving and nurturing hug. Feel the warmth and comfort of this embrace as you offer your inner child the love and care they deserve.

As we come to the end of this meditation, take a deep breath in, and slowly exhale. Remember that you are capable of being the healthy adult your inner child needs, offering them the love, care, and validation they deserve. Carry this feeling of connection and compassion with you throughout your day and your journey toward healing.

Reflect on any thoughts or feelings that arose during the meditation with the group. Remember to focus on both process and content. Use the following discussion questions:

- Did anyone have difficulty accessing their inner child? What got in the way?
- What was it like for you to say the affirmations to your inner child? Did any of them resonate with you or your inner child?
- Can you think of different affirmations that resonate with you or your inner child? What did your inner child need to hear to feel safe?

### Facilitators' Forum

To support group members in this process, consider suggesting they bring a picture of themselves as a child to the group session. This visual aid can help them connect more easily with their younger selves, triggering memories and emotions associated with that time.

Encourage group members to look into their eyes in the picture and reflect on the memory it represents. As they visualize themselves as a child, invite them to consider how they may have felt during that time. This additional layer of connection can deepen their engagement with the meditation and enhance their ability to access their inner child.

Engaging one's inner child can be challenging for some group members, especially those who have experienced childhood trauma or adverse childhood experiences. In that case, you can ask them to think of another child, not themselves, who they want to feel cared for and valued. Create a safe and supportive environment for them to share or refrain from sharing, respecting their boundaries and personal comfort levels.

### Activity 5.9 – Tuning In: Exploring Internal Cues in Eating Disorder Recovery

Research has suggested poor interoception, the ability to perceive and respond to internal bodily sensations, is associated with body image concerns and disordered eating patterns.[13] Interoceptive signals guide our eating behaviors, but impaired sensitivity to these signals naturally prevents one from responding to their needs. Factors contributing to impaired interoceptive sensitivity and awareness include pressure to be thin, focus on body shape and appearance, restrained eating, and weight stigma. Instead of honoring internal responses, these can lead to focusing on external methods, such as calorie counting or strict diets.[14] In short, body trust is lost.

It is essential for dietitians and therapists to acknowledge the challenges individuals with eating disorders face in recognizing and responding to their internal cues. Disordered eating behaviors often involve a disconnection between the body and mind, hindering individuals' ability to understand and prioritize their physiological and emotional needs.

The following discussion is meant to assist group members in developing this trust by better understanding their internal cues and learning (or relearning) to recognize, respect, and respond to them.

### Materials:

- For either in-person or virtual groups, a paper and pen may be needed if group members choose a journaling option (refer to activity instructions).

**Begin** by highlighting the significance of listening to and responding to internal cues as they help one recognize their physiological and emotional needs, which are essential for caring for themselves. Encourage group members to identify their own internal cues.

Offer examples:

- Hunger and fullness sensations
- Feeling satisfied and satiated
- Thirst and hydration needs
- Fatigue and sleepiness
- Emotional and stress-related responses
- Energy levels and activity needs
- Feeling too hot or too cold
- Urge to use the bathroom
- Sensory input, such as feeling overwhelmed by noise or crowds
- Feeling emotionally overwhelmed or anxious
- Feeling physically uncomfortable or in pain
- Feeling a sense of pleasure or enjoyment in certain activities

**Invite** group members to consider how they can identify their internal states and needs. For example, ask *How can you tell when you need to go to bed? What are the signs that indicate you are satiated after a meal?*

**Explain** how eating disorders, anxiety, and feelings of inadequacy can make it challenging to tune into and honor internal cues. These conditions can cause individuals to override or ignore their bodily signals, leading to disordered eating behaviors or other unhealthy coping mechanisms.

Ask the prompt:

> What factors can get in the way of being aware of and responsive to your body's needs? Some examples may include work or school deadlines, changes in sleep patterns, stress, perfectionism, rigid beliefs, and strict rules.

**Give** group members five minutes and a choice between journaling, sitting quietly with their thoughts, or doing a quick body scan to check in with how they are feeling physically and emotionally at that moment. Ask them to pay attention to their internal cues and practice mindfulness as they engage with themselves.

**Discuss** how practicing mindfulness and other techniques can help group members learn to better recognize and respond to their internal cues. Encourage group members to set aside time each day to reflect on how they feel physically and emotionally.

### Facilitators' Forum

The importance of setting boundaries to honor internal cues cannot be overstated. Facilitators could ask group members to identify areas in their lives where they may need to set boundaries to prioritize their physical and emotional well-being.

Examples could include setting limits on work hours or commitments, saying no to social events when feeling overwhelmed, or setting aside time for self-care activities.

### The Role of Assertive Communication in Eating Disorder Recovery

Individuals with eating disorders often face challenges in effectively communicating their needs, thoughts, and emotions. This lack of assertiveness is a characteristic trait of eating disorders and can contribute to developing and persisting eating disorder symptoms.[15] Notably, a 2013 study published in *European Psychiatry* revealed that low assertiveness, characterized by difficulties in expressing one's needs and advocating for oneself, is associated with increased severity of eating disorder behaviors and poorer treatment outcomes among individuals with eating disorders.[16]

Assertiveness training has shown promising effects on individuals with eating disorders, specifically in improving emotion regulation, reducing symptom severity, and decreasing the frequency of symptoms.[17] By developing assertiveness skills, individuals may be able to communicate their needs more effectively to others, seek support, and access necessary resources for their recovery. Assertive communication also provides a healthier alternative to expressing emotions, as individuals can express themselves directly and assertively without resorting to harmful behaviors or disordered eating patterns.

Another important aspect is the ability to build and maintain meaningful relationships. By expressing themselves assertively, individuals can establish open and honest connections with others, fostering understanding, trust, and support in their recovery process.

However, certain barriers can hinder assertive communication in eating disorder recovery. Individuals with low self-esteem may believe they are unworthy of love, help, or healing, leading them to withhold their needs and suppress their voices. Perfectionists may struggle to acknowledge their limitations and resist asking for assistance, assuming they should handle everything independently.

Additionally, individuals who have never learned effective communication skills may struggle to express themselves assertively. If they have experienced environments where it was unsafe or encouraged to withhold their needs, it can further impede their ability to communicate assertively.

Furthermore, some individuals may excessively focus on regulating the emotions of others, prioritizing others' needs over their own and neglecting to assert their desires and boundaries. It is important to overcome these barriers and develop assertiveness skills to advocate for oneself and facilitate a supportive environment for recovery.

## Activity 5.10: Setting Boundaries with Self and Others

This activity delves into the importance of setting healthy boundaries in eating disorder recovery. By practicing assertive communication, group members can establish a sense of control, identify triggers, and prioritize their wants and needs.

## Materials:

- For in-person groups, a bowl or basket, pen and paper are needed.
- Virtual groups will utilize a chat feature (no other materials needed).

**Introduce** the concept of assertiveness. Begin by providing a brief educational overview of assertiveness using the previous psychoeducation. Explain that assertiveness is a communication style that allows individuals to express their thoughts, feelings, and needs directly and respectfully.

**Emphasize** that assertiveness differs from aggression (being overly forceful) or passivity (being submissive). Share examples of assertive communication in everyday life to illustrate its effectiveness.

**Ask** group members to write down a scenario where they struggle to communicate assertively in the context of their eating disorder recovery. Encourage them to focus on situations like setting boundaries with family members around triggering topics or asking for accommodations in social situations (i.e., ensuring there is a plan for meals on a vacation). For virtual groups: Instruct group members to send their scenarios directly to the facilitators via a chat feature.

**Collect** the written scenarios and place them in a bowl in the center of the group.

**Pass** the bowl around, allowing each group member to randomly select a scenario someone else wrote. For virtual groups, group facilitators will "assign" each group member a scenario at random.

**Give** the group members time to brainstorm assertive responses to the selected scenarios. Encourage them to think about using "I" statements, setting clear boundaries, and considering the potential consequences of their response.

**Provide** the group with a sample assertiveness script (in the following dark box) as a guide. Explain that this script can be a starting point for their assertive responses. Share an example of modifying the script to fit their specific scenario. Encourage group members to personalize the script according to their own communication style and needs.

> "I feel [emotion] when [specific behavior or situation] because [explain impact]. In order to [state your needs or boundaries], I would appreciate it if [request or suggestion]."

**Invite** each group member to share the scenario they selected (or were assigned) and the assertive response they came up with.

**Facilitate** a conversation where group members can provide support, feedback, and suggestions for refining their assertiveness skills. Use the following discussion questions, if desired:

- How do you feel about setting boundaries with others? Do you tend to prioritize their needs over your own? What factors contribute to this tendency?
- Reflect on a time when you successfully set a boundary with someone during your eating disorder recovery. What strategies did you use to assert your needs effectively? How did it impact your relationship with that person?
- In what ways can setting boundaries with yourself positively impact your recovery journey? How can you hold yourself accountable while still being compassionate toward yourself?
- Share an experience where you encountered resistance or pushback when trying to set a boundary. How did you handle the situation? What lessons did you learn from that experience?
- What self-care practices can you engage in to support yourself when setting and maintaining boundaries becomes challenging? How can you nurture your emotional well-being during this process?
- Discuss the importance of self-awareness in setting boundaries. How can understanding your limits, values, and needs empower you to communicate assertively?

### Facilitators' Forum

The fear of judgment or rejection from others based on their appearance or the size of their body can inhibit individuals with eating disorders from asserting themselves or standing up for their needs. Occupying physical and emotional space without fear or guilt is an important aspect of recovery for individuals with eating disorders. It involves developing a sense of self-acceptance, assertiveness, and a healthy relationship with one's body and emotions.

## Notes

1  Gentry, J. Eric. 2002. "Compassion Fatigue." *Journal of Trauma Practice* 1 (3–4): 48. https://doi.org/10.1300/j189v01n03_03.
2  Myers, Shannon B., Alison C. Sweeney, Victoria Popick, Kimberly Wesley, Amanda Bordfeld, and Randy Fingerhut. 2012. "Self-Care Practices and Perceived Stress Levels among Psychology Graduate Students." *Training and Education in Professional Psychology* 6 (1): 56. https://doi.org/10.1037/a0026534.
3  Dorociak, Katherine E., Patricia A. Rupert, Fred B. Bryant, and Evan Zahniser. 2017. "Development of a Self-Care Assessment for Psychologists." *Journal of Counseling Psychology* 64 (3): 325–334. https://doi.org/10.1037/cou0000206.

4  Mallorquí-Bagué, Núria, Cristina Vintró-Alcaraz, Isabel Sánchez, Nadine Riesco, Zaida Agüera, Roser Granero, Susana Jiménez-Múrcia, José M. Menchón, Janet Treasure, and Fernando Fernández-Aranda. 2017. "Emotion Regulation as a Transdiagnostic Feature among Eating Disorders: Cross-Sectional and Longitudinal Approach." *European Eating Disorders Review* 26 (1): 53–61. https://doi.org/10.1002/erv.2570.

5  Treasure, Janet, and Ulrike Schmidt. 2013. "The Cognitive-Interpersonal Maintenance Model of Anorexia Nervosa Revisited: A Summary of the Evidence for Cognitive, Socio-Emotional and Interpersonal Predisposing and Perpetuating Factors." *Journal of Eating Disorders* 1 (1). https://doi.org/10.1186/2050-2974-1-13.

6  Neff, Kristin D. 2016. "Erratum to: The Self-Compassion Scale Is a Valid and Theoretically Coherent Measure of Self-Compassion." *Mindfulness* 7 (4): 1009. https://doi.org/10.1007/s12671-016-0560-6.

7  Kirschner, Hans, Willem Kuyken, Kim Wright, Henrietta Roberts, Claire Brejcha, and Anke Karl. 2019. "Soothing Your Heart and Feeling Connected: A New Experimental Paradigm to Study the Benefits of Self-Compassion." *Clinical Psychological Science* 7 (3): 545–565. https://doi.org/10.1177/2167702618812438.

8  Breines, Juliana, Aubrey Toole, Clarissa Tu, and Serena Chen. 2013. "Self-Compassion, Body Image, and Self-Reported Disordered Eating." *Self and Identity* 13 (4): 432–448. https://doi.org/10.1080/15298868.2013.838992.

9  Braun, Tosca D., Park, Crystal L., and Amy Gorin. 2016. "Self-Compassion, Body Image, and Disordered Eating: A Review of the Literature." *Body Image* 17: 117–131. Accessed June 27, 2023. https://doi.org/10.1016/j.bodyim.2016.03.003.

10  Tribole, Evelyn, and Elyse Resch. 2020. *Intuitive Eating: A Revolutionary Anti-Diet Approach.* New York: St. Martin's Essentials.

11  Kristeller, Jean L., Ruth A. Baer, and Ruth Quillian-Wolever. 2006. "Mindfulness-Based Approaches to Eating Disorders." *Mindfulness-Based Treatment Approaches*: 75–91. https://doi.org/10.1016/b978-012088519-0/50005-8.

12  Neff, Kristin. 2003. "Self-Compassion: An Alternative Conceptualization of a Healthy Attitude toward Oneself." *Self and Identity* 2 (2): 85–101. https://doi.org/10.1080/15298860309032.

13  Quadt, Lisa, Hugo D. Critchley, and Sarah N. Garfinkel. 2018. "The Neurobiology of Interoception in Health and Disease." *Annals of the New York Academy of Sciences* 1428 (1): 112–128. https://doi.org/10.1111/nyas.13915.

14  Quadt et al., "The Neurobiology of Interoception," 112–128.

15  Atti, Anna-Rita, Bandini, L., Valente, S., Sighinolfi, C., Mastellari, T., et al. 2019. "Cognitive-Behavioral Therapy for Group Assertive Training in Outpatients with Eating Disorders: An Open Label Trial." *Neural Plasticity and Clinical Practice* 2 (1): 1–8. https://doi.org/10.31579/NPCP.2019/007.

16  Bandini, L., Sighinolfi, C., Menchetti, M., Morri, M., De Ronchi, D., and Atti, A. R. 2013. "1111 – Assertiveness and Eating Disorders: The Efficacy of a CBT Group Training. Preliminary Findings." *European Psychiatry* 28: 1. https://doi.org/10.1016/s0924-9338(13)76215-1.

17  Atti et al., "Cognitive-Behavioral Therapy," 2019.

# Appendix 5A – Exploring the Function of My Eating Disorder (for Activity 5.2)

*Instructions*: Consider the following functions an eating disorder may serve. Circle the ones that apply to you. Note that some of them may overlap or be closely related to one another. Next, examine some of the functions circled using the following questions.

| Coping with difficult emotions (e.g., regulating emotions) | Gaining a sense of control over life | Avoiding discomfort or distress | Punishing yourself for perceived failures or shortcomings |
|---|---|---|---|
| Coping with feelings of shame or guilt | Numbing or distracting oneself from difficult emotions or memories | Managing stress or pressure | Coping with changes or transitions in life (e.g., fear of becoming an adult, divorce) |
| Fitting in with a particular social group or culture | Coping with feelings of loneliness or isolation | Maintaining a sense of identity or self-worth | Gaining feelings of competence or superiority over others |
|  | Feeling a sense of safety or security | Seeking validation or attention from others |  |

Function: _____

Could be addressed in other ways such as: _____, _____,

_____

Does my need for this function to be satisfied change as I develop a stronger sense of Self? If so, how?

_____

_____

_____

Function: _____

Could be addressed in other ways such as: _____, _____,

_____

Does my need for this function to be satisfied change as I develop a stronger sense of Self? If so, how?

_____

_____

_____

Function: _____

Could be addressed in other ways such as: _____, _____,

_____

Does my need for this function to be satisfied change as I develop a stronger sense of Self? If so, how?

_____

_____

_____

# Appendix 5B – Adventures in Self-Care (for Activity 5.3)

| Activities I Am Comfortable Practicing | Activities I Want to Try but Have Not Yet | Activities I Want to Try but Feel Afraid or Am Avoiding |
|---|---|---|
| • | • | • |
| • | • | • |
| • | • | • |
| • | • | • |
| • | • | • |

# Appendix 5C – Nurturing Self-Care in Eating Disorder Recovery (for Activity 5.5)

Self-care is an essential component of your healing during eating disorder recovery. This worksheet is designed to support you in exploring and embracing meaningful self-care practices. Remember to approach yourself with patience and compassion as you engage with these exercises, allowing yourself the time and space needed to cultivate a healthier and more loving relationship with yourself.

| | | |
|---|---|---|
| **Physical Self-Care** | Consider how you can physically care for yourself, promoting a healthy mind and body. Examples may include nourishing meals, engaging in gentle exercise, getting sufficient rest, or prioritizing relaxation.<br>Write down at least three ways you can show kindness and care for your physical well-being: | •<br>•<br>• |
| **Emotional Self-Care** | Reflect on the practices that nurture your emotional and mental well-being. These practices may include engaging in therapy, practicing self-compassion, journaling, engaging in creative outlets, or setting boundaries.<br>Identify three ways you can prioritize your emotional and mental health: | •<br>•<br>• |
| **Spiritual Self-Care** | Explore activities that connect you with your inner self and promote spiritual well-being. These endeavors may involve spending time in nature, practicing mindfulness or meditation, exploring personal values, or engaging in activities that bring peace and purpose.<br>List three ways you can cultivate your spiritual well-being: | •<br>•<br>• |

# Appendix 5D – Unpacking Vacation (for Activity 5.6)

| Vacation Action or Habit | What words describe this action or habit or encompass how you felt while doing it? | What are things that I could do more often to feel this way? | What can I do between now and the next group to practice this? |
|---|---|---|---|
| *Example: Reading before bed* | *At peace Drifting Quiet* | *Stretching Guided imagery meditations More reading Listening to music* | *Read for 10 minutes every night* |
| | | | |
| | | | |
| | | | |

# Chapter 6

# Unveiling Authenticity

## Exploring Identity and Values Beyond Eating Disorders

This chapter addresses the fundamental questions, "*Who am I without my eating disorder?*" and "*What are my values?*" Within the framework of therapeutic approaches, including Acceptance and Commitment Therapy (ACT), Motivational Interviewing (MI), Cognitive Behavioral Therapy (CBT), Solution-Focused Brief Therapy (SFBT), expressive therapies, and interpersonal theories, a range of group activities and discussions are presented. Each is designed to help group members recognize the misalignment between their eating disorder and their authentic values.

Through self-reflection and exploration, group discussions and activities aim to empower group members to transcend their eating disorders and discover their identities. By engaging in these activities, participants can uncover the dissonance between what truly matters to them, and the realities perpetuated by their eating disorders, which often contradict their core values. Participants are encouraged to go beyond the confines of their eating disorders and embrace a broader understanding of their identity for a renewed sense of purpose and authenticity.

## Eating Disorders and Identity: Unraveling the Complexities

Asking the question, "*Who are you without an eating disorder?*" can evoke feelings of unease and uncertainty. The eating disorder may have become so deeply intertwined with one's sense of self that it blurs the boundaries between the individual and the illness. Discerning where the person ends and where the disorder begins can become challenging. This over-identification with the illness is understandable, especially for those whose eating disorders developed during their formative years and persisted for decades. The eating disorder may have initially emerged as a response to emotional pain, serving to soothe, numb, express, or communicate that pain.

Moreover, certain eating disorders, such as Anorexia Nervosa (AN), can seemingly align with personal values of discipline, control, perfectionism, and

DOI: 10.4324/9781003430964-9

conformity to society's ideal of thinness. As a result, the eating disorder becomes ego-syntonic, meaning it becomes integrated into one's sense of self.

Early psychodynamic theorists recognized the association between identity disturbances and eating disorders, viewing them as disorders of the self. These theorists conceptualize the symptoms of an eating disorder as manifestations of inner turmoil, with disordered eating acting as a means for communicating underlying issues.[1] These behaviors can regulate emotions and interpersonal relationships and provide a sense of self-worth and agency.[2] The eating disorder may fulfill psychological needs for autonomy, competence, and control, ultimately becoming integral to a person's identity.[3]

While some individuals may take pride in their eating disorders, it is a source of shame for others. Regardless, because the behaviors are so entrenched, there is a tendency to perceive them as defining characteristics of a person rather than recognizing them as coping mechanisms developed over time. Well-intentioned clinicians seeking to alleviate their patient's eating disorder symptoms may inadvertently threaten that individual's sense of self.[4] Therefore, it is crucial to uncover a nuanced understanding of self, distinct from eating disorder behavior, to facilitate the process of recovery.

Through the exploration in this chapter, group members can discover their unique strengths and embrace the potential for personal growth and fulfillment. This process involves acknowledging group members' emotional attachment to the disorder while recognizing that it does not define who they are as individuals.

### Activity 6.1 – A Few of My Favorite Things

Encouraging group members to identify positive experiences or memories allows them to acknowledge aspects of themselves beyond their eating disorder. It is also a way for group members to get to know each other better and develop a greater sense of connection to themselves and each other.

### Materials:

- For in-person groups, provide paper and writing utensils for group members.
- For virtual groups, members can gather their writing materials or utilize electronic devices for the activity.

**Start** by allocating a few minutes for each group member to make a list of some of their favorite things by asking the prompt:

Take a few minutes to list some of your favorite things. They can be physical or experiential. The only caveat is that these should have nothing to do with your eating disorder.

**Allow** time for group members to contemplate the prompt and make a list. If the group needs help getting started, facilitators could give examples such as a cozy throw blanket, a cool breeze on an autumn morning, or a favorite article of clothing. Further the discussion by asking:

- Did you observe any changes in your body language, such as relaxed shoulders, softened breath, or a smile, as you made your list? If so, can you share what you noticed and how you felt?
- Did making your list trigger any particular memories or emotional experiences? If so, describe.
- Did you find it challenging to think about these things? If so, what do you think made it difficult?
- Do your answers reveal anything about your personality or sense of self?

**Encourage** group members to recognize shared interests or experiences and ask follow-up questions to one another. Doing so promotes a sense of camaraderie and support within the group, fostering connections beyond their eating disorder and facilitating a positive group dynamic.

### Facilitators' Forum

For some group members, asking them to identify their favorite things may feel too broad and could need to be simplified. Members who are perfectionistic and rigid in their thinking may overthink this prompt and second-guess themselves.

While limiting the allotted time to form the list can help prevent overthinking, facilitators can also ask direct questions or prompts as an alternative. Here are some suggestions:

- What is one of your favorite vacation memories?
- What is one of your favorite childhood memories?
- What is one of your favorite bands or types of music?
- What is one of your favorite scents?
- What is something that makes you smile?
- Share with the group a talent or skill that you possess.
- Share with the group something that may surprise them about you.

## Activity 6.2 – Life Through My Lens

Photography as a therapeutic tool is associated with improved emotional, cognitive, and expressive abilities at the individual and group levels. It promotes the ability to recognize and express an emotional experience without the limitations of verbal communication, which can lead to increased insight, self-awareness, and understanding.[5] The following exercise focuses not on the technical proficiency of the photographs but on the group member being present and capturing something meaningful to them.

Facilitators will introduce this exercise as "homework," tasking group members to take five pictures of things that are meaningful to them that they will share in the next group. Let them know this could be a picture of objects, even photographs, places, food, or people. Explain that the photo can be a metaphor or symbol of something important in their life now or something they would like to be significant in the future. Facilitators will instruct participants to avoid capturing images associated with their eating disorders. Group members are encouraged to be imaginative while also cautioned against overthinking.

This activity allows group members to rediscover or establish a sense of self separate from their eating disorder. It will enable them to shift their focus away from the illness and toward their strengths, interests, and passions. By consciously abstaining from documenting their eating disorder-related experiences, they can begin to reclaim their individuality and reshape their identity beyond the constraints of the disorder.

This process may involve exploring various aspects of their lives, such as hobbies, relationships, achievements, or personal growth. Group members can use this exercise to express themselves, emphasizing the positive elements of their lives that their eating disorders have overshadowed. Through this exploration, they may discover new facets of themselves and reconnect with aspects they may have neglected or forgotten.

Consciously refraining from capturing images related to their eating disorder can also foster a sense of empowerment, promoting a shift in perspective as it asks group members to view themselves as whole individuals rather than defined solely by their struggles. It allows group members to take control of their narrative and redefine themselves on their terms. By focusing on their unique qualities and experiences outside of the eating disorder, they can challenge the dominant role that the illness has played in their lives and explore and celebrate their identity beyond the illness.

## Materials:

- For both in-person and virtual groups, each member will need access to a camera, such as one on a smartphone or cellular phone.
- Group members or facilitators may print or present the pictures electronically.

Share the following prompt:

> Over the upcoming week, capture five pictures that hold personal significance to you. These images will be a way to share meaningful aspects of your life with the group.

**Request** participants share their photographs by emailing them directly to the facilitators or, for virtual groups, displaying them on their screen when asked to do so. In an in-person group, members can bring printed copies if preferred.

**Proceed** by allowing each group member to share their photographs and the significance behind them.

**Further** the conversation with open-ended questions encouraging reflection and discussion:

- How did you decide which photos to capture? Can you share your thought process and any considerations that influenced your choices?
- As you viewed the photographs shared by other group members, did you notice any recurring themes or patterns? What stood out to you and why?
- Reflecting on your experience with this exercise, what did you discover about yourself? Did it bring up any significant memories or emotions? If so, which ones?
- By viewing and discussing each other's photographs, what insights did you gain about each other? How may these insights contribute to your sense of connection as a group?

### Facilitators' Forum

Facilitators can modify the prompt to align the activity with a particular theme or focus. For example, if the group is exploring body functionality, the prompt could be to capture images that celebrate and appreciate different aspects of their bodies separate from appearance.

Another option is using photo prompts for specific emotions. Instead of capturing images of meaningful things, facilitators can ask participants to take photos representing particular emotions or moods. For example, facilitators could task group members with capturing images that evoke joy, serenity, resilience, or gratitude.

## From Struggle to Strength: Using Strengths in Recovery

The question of identity becomes complex and elusive when entangled with an eating disorder. It is common to swiftly identify what one is not, focusing on perceived shortcomings and failures. The brain is wired to prioritize problems, weaknesses, and negative or unfavorable circumstances.[6] This hardwiring can be traced back to our evolutionary development, where early humans needed to identify potential threats for survival. Those more attuned to danger had a better chance of staying alive and passing on their genes. Consequently, the human brain developed a tendency to prioritize negative information as a means of self-preservation, and this trait remains ingrained in our genetic makeup today.

The eating disorder, for many, becomes a way to protect themselves from real or perceived harm. It convinces them that they need it to be accepted, loved, or even to survive. Using strengths, professionals in psychology, specifically Positive Psychology, have discovered efficient and effective methods for assisting patients in connecting with their positive qualities, confronting challenges with resilience, and pursuing life objectives by leveraging their strengths. Ultimately, this approach enables greater self-awareness, elucidating questions of personal identity and harnessing their positive attributes to achieve personal growth and well-being.[7] When participants recognize their strengths, they can think about who they are apart from their eating disorder and use these strengths to empower them in their recovery.

## Activity 6.3 – Character Strength Exploration

This activity utilizes the classification of positive characteristics, referred to as the VIA Character Strengths, which emerged from the collaborative work of fifty-five scientists who conducted a comprehensive examination of psychological, philosophical, and theological literature. They aimed to identify, categorize, and measure universally valued positive qualities.[8],[9] There are multitudes of ways to use these strengths in group work. Group facilitators are encouraged to visit the VIA Institute of Character's website for more information, including links to research supporting strength identification in treating psychological distress.

## Materials:

- Worksheet "VIA Institute on Character's Classification of 24 Character Strengths" (Appendix 6A)
- For in-person groups, facilitators can display this list on a whiteboard or distribute individual copies to the participants.
- For virtual groups, either share a copy of the list with the participants via email before the group session or display it using screen share.

**Introduce** the VIA strengths list to the group using "VIA Institute on Character's Classification of 24 Character Strengths" (Appendix 6A), explaining that it lists twenty-four positive qualities identified through research as being universally valued across cultures.[10]

**Encourage** group members to choose three strengths from the list that resonate the most with them. Prompt group members:

> Looking at the list of character strengths, choose three that resonate with you. These strengths should make you think *"That's me,"* even if you don't always act in ways that demonstrate that strength.

**Ask** each member to share one or two of their strengths with the group. Encourage them to share a brief story or example of how they have used that strength.

**Proceed** by asking members to identify strengths that are particularly helpful in their eating disorder recovery. Some examples of relevant strengths might include the following:

- Self-regulation: Involves controlling impulses, delaying gratification, and modulating emotional responses.
- Gratitude: The ability to appreciate the good things in one's life, even amid struggles.
- Hope: The belief that circumstances can improve, even in the face of adversity.

**Ask** each group member to share a specific action they can take to cultivate one of those strengths in their life. For example, someone who wants to develop the strength of gratitude might commit to writing down three things they are grateful for each day.

**Emphasize** that overcoming an eating disorder is a gradual process that is often not linear. Facilitators should encourage group members to acknowledge each step toward enhancing one's strengths and celebrate it as progress.

### Facilitators' Forum

In a group familiar with the concept of diet culture, which will be thoroughly addressed in Chapter 8, facilitators can further the discussion by asking group members to consider what character strengths are celebrated in diet culture. How did these compare to those they identified as important in eating disorder recovery? Discussing how diet culture has dramatically co-opted self-regulation and perseverance as a "strength" can yield a fruitful conversation.

## The Use of Values to Facilitate Change

Values are concepts or ideals that hold significant meaning or importance for individuals.[11] By uncovering personally held values incompatible with their eating disorder behaviors (for example, placing importance on friendship and spending time with friends yet avoiding social situations involving food), individuals may be able to see how overarching personal values are compromised by their disorder.

Developing discrepancy, a tool in MI that is an intervention directed at improving motivation for behavioral change, is thought to be useful in treating eating disorders since a hallmark of the illness is the conflict between getting better and maintaining the eating disorder.[12]

By facilitating recognition or amplifying the discrepancy between eating disorder behavior and personal values or goals, group members begin to see how if they want to live a life truly aligned with their core values, one with meaning and fulfillment, it is necessary to move away from eating disorder behaviors. Facilitators can utilize values interventions to increase the motivation and willingness to feel discomfort that will arise in changing behavior that serves as a coping mechanism.

## Developing Willingness Using Values

Developing willingness is key to recovery from an eating disorder. It involves learning to accept difficult feelings and thoughts instead of suppressing them. ACT does not look to eliminate distressing thoughts, experiences, and feelings but instead promotes reconceptualizing and accepting them.[13] These feelings are expected when blocking urges to use symptoms that once may have provided a sense of control, soothing, self-worth, and reduced emotional pain, at least in the short term.

The primary goal of increasing willingness is to foster behavioral flexibility to enable behavior consistent with one's true values instead of being constrained by a behavior pattern maintained by a compulsion to avoid distress. The outcome is a more valued and meaningful life.[14] In service to one's values, a willingness may develop to feel the discomfort inherent in eating disorder recovery.

Facilitators have numerous ways to assist members in recognizing their values. They can use lists of values, card sorts, prompting questions, guided imagery, creative expression (such as collages), and more. We have picked a few of our favorites for the following activities. These activities attempt to increase members' clarity about what they truly value, examine how the eating disorder conflicts with these values, and help members identify actions to take concrete steps to live more in alignment with their true selves.

## Discussion 6.1: Tell Me About Your Hero

Getting members to think about what they value apart from appearance and external measures of success can be challenging in a society that treats weight loss as an accomplishment and what they can produce as more valuable than who they are. One way to elicit the identification of values is to prompt bigger-picture thinking. The "*at the end of the day, what is truly important*" type of questions are a creative way to accomplish this.

This discussion works best when facilitators do not give the goals and objectives at the outset. By refraining from explicitly stating the purpose of the activity, participants have the opportunity to discover that focusing on their body and food is less important than their eating disorder would have them believe. It opens space for exploring their values and identities separate from the eating disorder.

**Invite** group members to take a few minutes to think about someone they admire. This person could be someone they consider a hero or mentor. Someone who has inspired them in some way. Someone who has positively impacted their life. Someone they know personally or someone they have never met.

**Ask** the question:

Who is this person, and why did you choose them?
What qualities or traits in this person do you admire?

**Introduce** the following statements or variations of them to the group:

- "Hold on. I'm noticing something. As we've been sharing about the person we admire, I realized no one mentioned their weight or waist size. What does this observation tell you?"
- "Take a moment to reflect on this: weight or body size didn't come up in all the qualities and traits we've discussed. What can we learn from this experience?"
- "Consider the absence of weight or body-related attributes in our admiration for others. How can this insight inform and support your recovery?"
- "Let us explore how this experience of focusing on non-appearance-related qualities can be a valuable lesson for your recovery. How can you use this realization to shape your mindset and relationship with your body?"

### Facilitators' Forum

If a participant admires the appearance of the person they chose, it offers an opportunity to discuss conditional acceptance and societal pressures related to appearance-based values. This discussion promotes a deeper understanding of the impact of appearance-focused values and encourages unconditional self-acceptance and appreciation of inner qualities. Emphasizing that individuals don't lose their worth as human beings when their bodies change, the activity challenges the notion that appearance defines inherent worth. Discussing the qualities and traits admired in others that extend beyond physical appearance allows participants to recognize the value of character, actions, and personal growth. This understanding promotes a more inclusive mindset, embracing intrinsic value irrespective of physical changes and appreciating the uniqueness and inner qualities that make each person valuable.

## Activity 6.4: Values Collage

Using creative expression may help some members identify their values through introspection and self-exploration. Collaging, song, poetry, and creative writing may convey emotions and unearth someone's values in a way that looking at lists of words cannot.

Creative expression is also dynamic, flexible, and imperfect. These qualities challenge the rigidity of the eating disorder and perfectionistic standards that some members may experience.

## Materials:

- For in-person groups, provide each member with a piece of paper or a poster board and various magazines, markers, and other materials to cut, paste, and draw onto their collage. They may also bring in items from home they may want to add to their collage, such as personal photographs, drawings, or other elements such as ticket stubs, objects found in nature, etc.
- For virtual groups, this can be given as homework or done in real-time. Ask members to use paper or poster board and materials like magazines and markers to cut, paste, and draw onto their collages. They may also add in other items, such as those mentioned earlier.

**Introduce** the concept of values and how they relate to eating disorders. Explain that values are the guiding principles that give our lives meaning and purpose.

**Present** the prompt:

> Consider your core values, such as honesty, compassion, creativity, spirituality, etc. Reflect on what truly matters to you and what you want to stand for.

**Instruct** group members to cut out words, phrases, and images that represent their values.

Remind them that these should be meaningful and even aspirational things, which may not align with how they are currently living their life. Allow plenty of time for the participants to work on their collages. Remind them that the process is more important than the final product and that there is no right or wrong way to do it.

**Allot** time for group members to share what they have created after they have completed their collages.

Encourage discussion by asking:

- What values are most important to you?
- How do these values relate to your eating disorder?
- How can you use these values to guide your recovery?

**Summarize** the activity by emphasizing the importance of connecting with their values and using them as a compass in their lives. Remind the group that recovery is not just about overcoming symptoms. It is also about finding a deeper sense of purpose and meaning group members cannot find within the confines of their eating disorder.

*Facilitators' Forum*

For in-person groups, facilitators can pre-select and provide materials for the collages that exclude triggering images and advertisements promoting unattainable body standards and diet culture messaging to create a safe and supportive environment. By curating a collection of pre-cut words and pictures, participants can focus on their creative expression and exploration of personal values and identities without the risk of encountering harmful or triggering content. The materials should reflect inclusivity, self-acceptance, diversity, body neutrality or positivity, and a wide range of interests, hobbies, and passions.

## Activity 6.5: Values Voyage

This values clarification exercise is adapted from the "Bull's Eye" activity by Dr. Russ Harris in his 2008 book *The Happiness Trap: How to Stop Struggling and Start Living*.[15] His version was an adaptation from the Bull's Eye Values Survey (BEVS).[16]

In this activity, facilitators will ask group members to examine the discrepancy between their values in several life domains and how closely they live by them. For example, a person with a binge eating disorder may value happiness and enjoy food, but their disorder causes them to feel out of control when it comes to eating, leading to feelings of shame and guilt. Similarly, a person with an eating disorder may hold certain values such as health, self-care, and social justice, but their behaviors and thoughts related to food and body image may directly conflict with those values.

Lastly, facilitators will ask participants to identify a committed action plan. This action plan is the commitment to make a behavioral or mindset-oriented change in service to something bigger and more meaningful than their eating disorder.

When engaging in value clarification exercises, facilitators should adopt a gradual approach. This is because exploring and clarifying personal values involves introspection that can be challenging to navigate all at once.[17] Participants can better manage the emotions and reflections that arise by taking it step by step. This activity may take several group sessions to complete, so it is divided into three parts, providing natural places for facilitators to pause and resume the activity as indicated.

## Materials:

- Worksheet "Values Voyage" (Appendix 6B)
- For in-person groups, provide paper and writing utensils for group members.
- For virtual groups, members can gather their writing materials or utilize electronic devices for the activity.

**Begin** this exercise by clarifying the difference between values and goals. Values are beliefs about things that are very important to us. They are principles group members stand for as opposed to items, like goals, that they can check off a list.

- Provide an example for clarification: To eat whatever the locals serve while traveling might be a goal; to be immersed and present, experiencing and honoring diversity and another's culture may be the underlying values.

### Part 1: Identifying Values in Life Domains

**Introduce** the seven identified domains in "Values Voyage" (Appendix 6B): intimate relationships, other family relationships, friendships, career, spirituality, community, and leisure.

**Ask** each group member to select one or two domain(s) to focus on.

### Part 2: Eating Disorder in the Way

**Further** group members to identify their values in their chosen domains using Part 2 of "Values Voyage (Appendix 6B)." Questions included on the worksheet are meant to help participants access the values in each domain.

**Ask** group members to look at how the eating disorder and its associated beliefs and behaviors appear in the domain(s) they chose. Encourage them to consider how these incongruencies interfere with living a life consistent with their values.

### Part 3: Committed Action

**Emphasize** that identifying their true values and aligning their behaviors with those values requires addressing the underlying psychological issues contributing to the disorder's development and maintenance. Exploring barriers to change is vital.

**Ask** group members: Can you identify one thing you are willing to do this week to move you closer to living in alignment with your values? Let them know that this would require making room for the thoughts, memories, feelings, sensations, and urges that come from not allowing those eating disorder beliefs to control them.

**Have** group members complete the following prompt and share it with the group (Part 3 of "Values Voyage" [Appendix 6B]):

In service to my value of _____. I am willing to
                          (*identify value(s)*)

_____.
(identify one step they are willing to take to change their behavior)

**Provide** accountability to any group members who would like the group's support. Specifically, suggest group members check in with how they did with their committed action in the next group session. To mitigate shame and bolster courage, reassure group members that it is normal to face challenges when making changes; there is no expectation that this will feel effortless.

### Facilitators' Forum

Although identifying values can help inform behavior and increase willingness to change and feel the associated discomfort, facilitators must assess the group members' current skills, which will be necessary to elicit that change. For instance, members may want to nurture friendships but lack the social skills needed. There also may be underlying trauma that can inform reactions that keep them from connecting with others. Values may increase the willingness to address this trauma.

Remind group members that the eating disorder results from a deeper psychological struggle, and the individual's true self often does not align with their disordered thoughts and behaviors.

## Discussion 6.2: If I Had Peace with Food and My Body

This activity is adapted from Solution-Focused Therapy's Miracle Question intervention and Dr. Russ Harris' book *The Confidence Gap: A Guide to Overcoming Fear and Self-Doubt*, specifically the ACT exercise that begins "*In a world where you had unlimited confidence . . .*"[18,19] The objectives of this activity include helping members gain insight and perspective into the acuity of their eating disorder, informing goals, clarifying values, and reconnecting them with what they want and who they truly are. This process can provide hope as they imagine a future without their eating disorder holding them back.

**Invite** group members to close their eyes if they are comfortable doing so and imagine the following:

Imagine waking up in the morning, and as you gradually become aware of your surroundings, you suddenly realize that you have completely recovered from your eating disorder. It feels like a dream, as you cannot recall how this transformation occurred. All you know is that something has shifted within you. You are finally at peace with food and your body. You no longer have intrusive thoughts about food or your body. You are experiencing the freedom you have not always believed was possible.

**Ask** members to open their eyes.

**Initiate** discussion using the following questions:

- How would getting up and getting dressed in the morning look different? How might it feel different?
- How would it impact your choices around food?
- How would you interact with people differently, be it your family, friends, or someone you are dating or interested in dating?
- How would your relationships change?
- How might you act differently at school or work?
- What might you try doing that you have avoided?
- What might you stop doing or do less of?
- How would you talk to yourself differently?
- Which qualities of your personality might become more evident?
- How would others know you recovered from your eating disorder?

**Check in** with group members regarding the process, not only the content of their answers. For example: *How was it for you trying to imagine being fully recovered from your eating disorder?* Make connections between members' responses, encourage them to do the same, and show excitement at the possibilities recovery may bring.

**Encourage** group members to share any observations or realizations about the conflict between their eating disorder and their true values, guiding the discussion toward promoting self-compassion and growth.

### Facilitators' Forum

Some members may find the idea of going to sleep and waking up recovered too much of a fantasy and too vague and therefore difficult to access. This ambiguity can lead group members to give superficial answers or not even attempt to respond to the prompt. Facilitators can use this prompt as an alternative:

> Picture a scenario where we unexpectedly come across each other. It could be at a park, a museum, or even a restaurant. As we run into each other, you greet me warmly, and I notice you smile. I ask how you have been, and you respond positively, mentioning that you are finally at peace with food and your body. I ask you to tell me more about how your life has changed. I let you know I want to hear all about it. I want to hear how things are different for you now. What sorts of things would you share with me?

## Discussion 6.3: Food Culture and Personal Values

Food often connects individuals to their family traditions, religious practices, or cultural heritage. However, those with eating disorders may struggle with allowing themselves to enjoy foods that are part of their customs, even if they value their cultural or religious identity. For example, someone identifying strongly with their religious heritage may use symptoms during holiday meals. Even those with deep family values may struggle with participating in family traditions involving food. In essence, the eating disorder interferes with the ability to fully experience and engage with these cultural and familial identities.

**Ask** the prompt:

> Reflect on a religious, cultural, or familial tradition that holds significance for you, particularly in relation to the food involved. Recall a specific instance when your eating disorder challenged your ability to enjoy and engage in that experience.

**Offer** examples if needed, such as restricting favorite foods on Christmas morning or compulsively exercising after a July 4th barbecue instead of visiting with loved ones.

**Encourage** participants to share their chosen experiences.

**Conclude** by emphasizing the significance of food as being intricately linked to memories, identity, and tradition. If desired, further the discussion by asking:

- How does the eating disorder interfere with these rituals or customs?
- Can this interference jeopardize an individual's value system and diminish the richness of these cherished identities? If so, how?
- How can you use this discovery to motivate you toward recovery?

### Facilitators' Forum

This activity will inevitably involve more food talk than other activities in this book. In addition to advancing the conversation using the previous discussion questions, the dietitian can challenge any uses of "bad" or "unhealthy" food language. Remind (or educate) group members about the concept of food neutrality and the importance of including foods in our diets in ways that feel fulfilling and satisfactory to each of us. How group members do that will look different to each person, and that is okay; there is no single "right" way to eat.

Mitigating the shame around the enjoyment of celebratory foods is important as well. Throughout history, food has been a prominent component of celebration and ritual. It makes sense that the foods that have sustained decades and centuries are ones that taste delicious and feel special. It is not wrong or shameful to enjoy them. It is in our nature.

Facilitators are encouraged to bring attention to the body language they notice and share these observations with the group members. For example, seeing that someone may smile when recalling a food that has held meaning to them or giving great detail about a food that is significant to their heritage are observations that may be valuable for the group to recognize.

## Notes

1  Bruch, Hilde. 1979. *Eating Disorders: Obesity, Anorexia Nervosa, and the Person within*. New York: Basic Books.
2  Amianto, Federico, Georg Northoff, Giovanni Abbate Daga, Secondo Fassino, and Giorgio A. Tasca. 2016. "Is Anorexia Nervosa a Disorder of the Self? A Psychological Approach." *Frontiers in Psychology* 7. https://doi.org/10.3389/fpsyg.2016.00849.
3  Froreich, Franzisca V., Lenny R. Vartanian, Matthew J. Zawadzki, Jessica R. Grisham, and Stephen W. Touyz. 2016. "Psychological Need Satisfaction, Control, and Disordered Eating." *British Journal of Clinical Psychology* 56 (1): 53–68. https://doi.org/10.1111/bjc.12120.
4  Bulik, Cynthia M., and Kenneth S. Kendler. 2000. " 'I Am What I (Don't) Eat': Establishing an Identity Independent of an Eating Disorder." *American Journal of Psychiatry* 157 (11): 1755–1760. https://doi.org/10.1176/appi.ajp.157.11.1755.
5  Saita, Emanuela, and Martina Tramontano. 2018. "Navigating the Complexity of the Therapeutic and Clinical Use of Photography in Psychosocial Settings: A Review of the Literature." *Research in Psychotherapy: Psychopathology, Process and Outcome*. https://doi.org/10.4081/ripppo.2018.293.
6  Baumeister, Roy F., Ellen Bratslavsky, Catrin Finkenauer, and Kathleen D. Vohs. 2007. "Bad Is Stronger than Good." *Review of General Psychology* 5 (4): 323–370. https://doi.org/10.1037/1089-2680.5.4.323.
7  Baumeister et al., "Bad is Stronger Than Good," 2007.
8  Peterson, Christopher, and Seligman Martin E. P. 2004. *Character Strengths and Virtues: A Handbook and Classification*. Washington, DC: American Psychological Association.
9  Dahlsgaard, Katherine, Christopher Peterson, and Martin E. Seligman. 2005. "Shared Virtue: The Convergence of Valued Human Strengths across Culture and History." *Review of General Psychology* 9 (3): 203–213. https://doi.org/10.1037/1089-2680.9.3.203.
10  Niemiec, Ryan M., and Ruth Pearce. 2021. "The Practice of Character Strengths: Unifying Definitions, Principles, and Exploration of What's Soaring, Emerging, and Ripe with Potential in Science and in Practice." *Frontiers in Psychology* 11. https://doi.org/10.3389/fpsyg.2020.590220.
11  Hayes, Steven C., Jason B. Luoma, Frank W. Bond, Akihiko Masuda, and Jason Lillis. 2006. "Acceptance and Commitment Therapy: Model, Processes and Outcomes." *Behaviour Research and Therapy* 44 (1): 1–25. https://doi.org/10.1016/j.brat.2005.06.006.
12  Weiss, Carmen V., Jennifer S. Mills, Henny A. Westra, and Jacqueline C. Carter. 2013. "A Preliminary Study of Motivational Interviewing as a Prelude to Intensive Treatment for an Eating Disorder." *Journal of Eating Disorders* 1 (1). https://doi.org/10.1186/2050-2974-1-34.
13  Hayes, Steven C., Kirk D. Strosahl, and Kelly G. Wilson. 2003. *Acceptance and Commitment Therapy: An Experiential Approach to Behavior Change*. London: Guilford Press.
14  Juarascio, Adrienne, Jena Shaw, Evan M. Forman, C. Alix Timko, James D. Herbert, Meghan L. Butryn, and Michael Lowe. 2013. "Acceptance and Commitment Therapy for Eating Disorders: Clinical Applications of a Group Treatment." *Journal of Contextual Behavioral Science* 2 (3–4): 85–94. https://doi.org/10.1016/j.jcbs.2013.08.001.

15 Harris, Russ. 2022. *The Happiness Trap: How to Stop Struggling and Start Living.* Boulder, CO: Shambhala.

16 Lundgren, Tobias, Jason B. Luoma, JoAnne Dahl, Kirk Strosahl, and Lennart Melin. 2012. "The Bull's-Eye Values Survey: A Psychometric Evaluation." *Cognitive and Behavioral Practice* 19 (4): 518–526. https://doi.org/10.1016/j.cbpra.2012.01.004.

17 Vyskocilova, J., Prasko, J., Ociskova, M., Sedlackova, Z., Marackova, M., Holubova, M., Hruby, R., and Slepecky, M. 2016. "Values and Values Work in Cognitive Behavioral Therapy." *European Psychiatry* 33 (S1): S456–S457. https://doi.org/10.1016/j.eurpsy.2016.01.1660.

18 Harris, Russ. *The Confidence Gap: A Guide to Overcoming Fear and Self-Doubt.* Boston: Trumpeter, 2011.

19 De Shazer, Steve, Insoo Kim Berg, Eve Lipchik, Elam Nunnally, Alex Molnar, Wallace Gingerich, and Michele Weiner-Davis. 1986. "Brief Therapy: Focused Solution Development." *Family Process* 25 (2): 207–221. https://doi.org/10.1111/j.1545-5300.1986.00207.x.

# Appendix 6A – VIA Institute on Character's Classification of 24 Character Strengths (for Activity 6.3)[1]

Table 6.1 The VIA Institute on Character's six domains and 24 character strengths.

| Wisdom | **Creativity** ✦ Clever ✦ Original & adaptive ✦ Problem solver<br>**Curiosity** ✦ Interested ✦ Explores new things ✦ Open to new ideas<br>**Judgment** ✦ Critical thinker ✦ Thinks things through ✦ Open-minded<br>**Love of Learning** ✦ Masters new skills and topics ✦ Systematically adds to knowledge<br>**Perspective** ✦ Wise ✦ Provides wise counsel ✦ Takes the big picture view |
|---|---|
| **Courage** | **Bravery** ✦ Shows valor ✦ Doesn't shrink from fear<br>**Perseverance** ✦ Persistent ✦ Industrious ✦ Finishes what one starts<br>**Honesty** ✦Authentic ✦ Trustworthy ✦ Sincere<br>**Zest** ✦ Enthusiastic ✦ Energetic ✦ Doesn't do things halfheartedly |
| **Humanity** | **Love** ✦ Warm and genuine ✦ Values close relationships<br>**Kindness** ✦ Generous ✦ Nurturing ✦ Caring ✦ Compassionate ✦ Altruistic<br>**Social Intelligence** ✦Aware of the motivates and feelings of self/others ✦ Knows what makes others tick |
| **Justice** | **Teamwork** ✦ Team player ✦ Socially responsible ✦ Loyal<br>**Fairness** ✦ Just ✦ Doesn't let feelings bias decisions about others<br>**Leadership** ✦ Organizes group activities ✦ Encourages a group to get things done |
| **Temperance** | **Forgiveness** ✦ Merciful ✦ Accepts' other's shortcomings ✦ Gives people a second chance<br>**Humility** ✦ Modest ✦ Let one's accomplishments speak for themselves<br>**Prudence** ✦ Careful ✦ Cautious ✦ Doesn't take undue risks<br>**Self-regulation** ✦ Self-controlled ✦ Disciplined ✦ Manages impulses and emotions |

| Transcendence | **Appreciation of Beauty & Excellence** ✦ Feels awe and wonder in beauty ✦ Inspired by goodness of others<br>**Gratitude** ✦ Thankful for the good ✦ Expresses thanks ✦ Feels blessed<br>**Hope** ✦ Optimistic ✦ Future-minded ✦ Future orientated<br>**Humor** ✦ Playful ✦ Brings smiles to others ✦ Lighthearted<br>**Spirituality** ✦ Searches for meaning ✦ Feels a sense of purpose ✦ Senses a relationship with the sacred |
|---|---|

## Note

1 "The 24 Character Strengths." VIA Institute on Character. www.viacharacter.org/character-strengths.

# Appendix 6B – "Values Voyage" (for Activity 6.5)

## Part 1: Domains

*Intimate relationships*: What type of individual would you like to be in an intimate relationship? To answer this, consider the behaviors you would like to exhibit in those relationships and the values that support those actions. Think about your underlying motives and how they align with the qualities you appreciate in a relationship. Focus on the value and avoid mentioning specific goals, i.e., marriage.

*Other family relationships*: This area of focus pertains to the nuclear family and your extended family. What type of relative do you want to be (such as a son/daughter, uncle/aunt, grandfather/grandmother, father-in-law/mother-in-law, etc.)? Reflect on the values you want to embody in this area of your life.

*Friendships*: What type of friend do you aspire to be? Reflect on the qualities of your closest friends and see if you can use those relationships to identify values that are important to you in this area.

*Career*: What kind of employee do you strive to be, regardless of whether your job is straightforward or highly specialized? What are your top priorities in your work, and what do you hope to accomplish in your career? What qualities are important for you to have or develop in that domain?

*Spirituality*: Spirituality is not limited to organized religion, although it is undoubtedly part of this area. Spirituality encompasses everything that fosters a sense of connection with something beyond oneself and evokes feelings of wonder or transcendence. What kind of person do you aspire to be in this aspect of your life?

*Community*: Think about your desire to contribute to society. What qualities do you want to bring to your role as a community member? Think about qualities you want to possess in social, political, charitable, and other related areas.

*Leisure*: Consider the significance of your hobbies, sports, games, trips, and other leisure activities. Reflect on the values you want to bring to these pursuits in your life. What draws you to that activity/interest? How do you want to feel when you are engaged in them? If they are important, why?

Select two domains to focus on: —————— & ——————

## Part 2: ED in the Way

Looking at your two selected domains, consider:

- What would you value if nothing was getting in your way (including barriers related to beliefs or rules about eating, food, and your body)?
- What is meaningful to you? What would you like to be meaningful?
- What qualities would you like to bring to these two domains?

Example:

---

Domain: *Friendships*
Values:
- *Connection*
- *Non-judgmental*
- *Empathetic*

Eating Disorder Incongruencies:
- *ED prevents me from feeling present, leads to feeling isolated*
- *ED leads to the judgment of self and others*
- *Numb to the needs of others, preoccupied with self*

---

Identify values in each area:

| *Domain 1:* | *Domain 2:* |
|---|---|
| Values: | Values: |
| • | • |
| • | • |
| • | • |
| • | • |
| • | • |
| Eating Disorder Incongruencies: | Eating Disorder Incongruencies: |
| • | • |
| • | • |
| • | • |

## Part 3: Commitment

Example:

In service to my value of connection, I am willing to say yes to an invitation to my friend's birthday dinner and eat birthday cake.

In service to my value of ————————————————, I am willing to
(identify value[s])

—————————————————————————————————————— .
(identify one step they are willing to take to change their behavior)

# Chapter 7

# Breaking Barriers

## Overcoming Resistance and Creating Lasting Change in Eating Disorder Recovery

When individuals engage in weight control behaviors, such as restrictive eating or compulsive exercise, they may experience temporary feelings of confidence or relief from distress. However, the long-term physical and emotional consequences for most outweigh any perceived benefits. Despite the desire to stop suffering and find peace with food and their bodies, fear leads to resisting change.

For many, the eating disorder has become intertwined with their identity, raising concerns about what will remain if fully recovered. They may fear being unable to manage the overwhelming emotions that surface when their coping mechanisms are no longer present. This chapter will address barriers to change in eating disorder recovery, including shame, guilt, perfectionism, and limiting beliefs, and offer strategies to overcome them.

There are several therapeutic approaches employed in this chapter. Cognitive Behavioral Therapy (CBT) principles are incorporated to challenge unhelpful patterns of thinking and behaviors. Acceptance and Commitment Therapy (ACT) techniques encourage participants to allow discomfort and pursue meaningful change aligned with their values. Self-compassion and expressive writing will help participants cultivate a compassionate inner voice. The activities and discussions in this chapter facilitate deeper exploration, self-efficacy, growth, and self-confidence to support group members in reclaiming their lives and finding peace and fulfillment beyond the confines of their eating disorders.

### Narrowing the Lens: The Impact of Eating Disorders on Quality of Life, Relationships, and Motivation for Change

Eating disorders profoundly impact a person's physical, psychological, and psychosocial functioning. A study investigating eating disorder patients' quality of life showed that patients with eating disorders presented with a significantly lower quality of life compared to the general population and those with mood disorders. Contrary to the commonly perceived diagnostic hierarchy discussed

DOI: 10.4324/9781003430964-10

in Chapter 3, the study results indicate no significant differences in the quality of life among the different eating disorder diagnostic groups.[1]

Individuals with eating disorders often experience intense anxiety and distress around food, body weight, and shape. They may struggle with low self-esteem, body image disturbances, and feelings of shame or guilt related to their eating disorder behaviors.

The impact of eating disorders extends beyond the individual and undoubtedly affects relationships with family, friends, coworkers, or classmates. Social activities that involve food can become stressful or triggering, leading to isolation and withdrawal. Individuals who consider themselves honest might lie to others to maintain their illness, jeopardizing trust in their relationships. Furthermore, the financial encumbrance of treatment and medical care can be substantial, adding to the stress and burden of living with an eating disorder.

Highlighting the degree to which the eating disorder narrows the ability to pursue other life goals is often helpful in increasing motivation to change eating disorder behaviors. By helping the participants identify what their eating disorder has cost them and clarifying what they truly want for their lives, researchers found they could increase their participants' willingness to undergo the challenging work needed to make behavioral changes.[2]

## Cognitive Flexibility and Its Role in Eating Disorder Recovery

Cognitive flexibility is fundamental to eating disorder recovery. Unlike the rigid and dichotomous thinking commonly found in individuals with eating disorders and comorbid conditions like Anxiety Disorders and Depressive Disorders, cognitive flexibility enables individuals to perceive shades of gray. This cognitive skill involves zooming out to recognize nuances and explore possibilities beyond the confines of the eating disorder's rules, mindsets, and unrealistic expectations. By cultivating cognitive flexibility, participants can discover alternative ways, other than using eating disorder symptoms, to meet their needs.

## Activity 7.1 – Shifting Perspective

This activity introduces the concept of viewing situations from different perspectives, encouraging a more flexible approach to thinking and behavior. By examining how events, or in this case, images, can be interpreted in various ways, participants are prompted to open up to new possibilities. The aim of this activity is to enhance group members' comprehension of the factors that shape their perceptions and subsequent behaviors, while simultaneously honing their cognitive restructuring skills.

To engage in this activity, facilitators will need a selection of ambiguous images. Ambiguous images possess an inherent vagueness that allows participants to construct diverse narratives from them. Their value is that the images' details do not unequivocally define the situation, leaving room for imaginative interpretations. For instance, envision a picture featuring four adults wearing concerned expressions, huddled around a piece of paper. This image lacks the contextual cues needed to determine whether these individuals are siblings poring over a will after the death of a parent or classmates reviewing their grade on a group assignment.

You can obtain these images from magazines, online sources, or even generate them using artificial intelligence software. Ambiguous images are not restricted to those containing people; they encompass a broad spectrum of subjects including landscapes, objects, abstract shapes, and more. The defining characteristic is that the image's content fosters multiple plausible interpretations.

Consider the following examples of ambiguous images:

- A Distant Horizon: A photograph depicting a hazy horizon where the sky meets the sea can evoke either a serene sunset scene or a misty morning on the beach, depending on the viewer's perspective.
- Crowded Street Corner: An image portraying a bustling street corner with people hurriedly moving could signify a busy urban scene during rush hour or a jubilant parade celebrating a local event.
- Elderly Couple: A photograph capturing an elderly couple seated together might convey a peaceful moment of companionship or a contemplative instance where one person consoles the other.
- Family Gathering: An image illustrating a family gathered around a table could be interpreted as a festive holiday meal or a solemn occasion where relatives unite in support.

**Begin** the activity by displaying an ambiguous image for the group. In virtual groups, facilitators can use a screen-sharing feature.

**Engage** the participants by asking them to share what they see in the picture and what story they believe the image tells. Encourage multiple interpretations and emphasize that there is no right or wrong answer.

**Facilitate** a discussion around the emotional responses evoked by different interpretations. Explore personal experiences, beliefs, biases, and individual perspectives contributing to varying interpretations. Encourage participants to consider the subjectivity of perception and how it can shape their understanding of a situation using the following questions as a guide:

- What do you see in this picture? What is the story?
- Do you notice having any emotional response to the picture when you hear different interpretations? If so, does your emotional response change depending on the interpretation?
- Why may some members look at the same picture and interpret it differently?

- Did any of these images evoke positive or negative feelings, and if so, how did those influence your perspective?
- What have you discovered through this exercise? How may it be relevant to your eating disorder or recovery?

**Explore** how rigid thought patterns associated with members' eating disorders can be challenged and transformed by adopting different perspectives.

### *Facilitators' Forum*

Support participants in making connections between their thoughts, emotions, and behaviors, emphasizing this essential principle of CBT. Group members may have acquired knowledge about this concept but need help to apply it effectively to overcome the rigid thought patterns associated with their eating disorders.

## Realistic Goals and Expectations

Having unrealistic goals and expectations related to the challenges participants may face can be a significant barrier to change. Perhaps a group member expects to never again have the urge to binge, purge, or restrict. Then when that urge comes, which it will, they feel discouraged and question the point of recovery. They may also lack the skills or experience to challenge their eating disorder behaviors, feeling disheartened when pursuing recovery is inevitably harder than imagined.

Setting realistic and attainable goals can significantly contribute to a person's sense of competence and efficacy during eating disorder recovery. Instead of setting overly broad objectives, focusing on making smaller, incremental changes can enhance feelings of mastery and foster a belief in one's ability to enact change.

Being successful in making changes requires participants to understand the barriers to making those changes. By setting well-crafted goals, individuals can enhance their clarity, motivation, and accountability, ultimately improving their chances of successful recovery. Sharing one's goal with the group or other supports may help increase accountability.

## Activity 7.2 – Enhancing Recovery Through SMART Goals

Individuals in eating disorder recovery are no strangers to goals. Goals are frequently set with outpatient providers and could include food-specific challenge goals, setting boundaries with friends or family members, or setting goals around symptom cessation.

A well-known goal-setting technique is setting SMART goals, developed by George T. Doran in 1981.[3] While the SMART (an acronym for Specific, Measurable, Achievable, Relevant, Time-Bound) format may receive criticism when applied to long-term goals, it proves valuable in this context as individuals with eating disorders benefit from concise, actionable, and short-term objectives. In part one of this activity, group members will learn how to apply SMART to their recovery. In part two, they will have the opportunity to practice using this tool.

## Materials:

- Worksheet "Setting SMART Goals" (Appendix 7A)
- For in-person groups, provide paper and writing utensils for group members.
- For virtual groups, members can gather their writing materials or utilize electronic devices for the activity.

### Part One

**Introduce** the SMART acronym and its components: Specific, Measurable, Achievable, Relevant, and Time-Limited. Describe how it can enhance recovery by helping group members set clear goals and stay focused on their progress.

**Discuss** each component, providing explanations and examples related to recovery from eating disorders:

- Specific: The goal should be clear, well-defined, and unambiguous. For example, instead of aiming for full recovery, a specific goal could be to eat a balanced breakfast seven days per week following a meal plan.
- Measurable: The goal must include criteria for tracking progress and determining when it is achieved. For example, maintaining a record or log of each occurrence of body-checking behaviors, such as pinching the stomach, can help monitor and measure progress.
- Achievable: The goal should be realistic and feasible. Instead of setting an unrealistic expectation of never body-checking again, it may be more achievable to identify a specific behavior to reduce, such as using a tape measure for body-checking.
- Relevant: The goal needs to be related to a larger goal, which in the group's case is recovery from the eating disorder. Willingness to feel discomfort increases when it is related to something meaningful and aligned with members' values; therefore, they may need to dig deeper and identify reasons for recovery.
- Time-Limited: The goal should have a designated time limit to maintain focus and prevent procrastination. Remember, the goal is a step in the recovery process – not recovery itself.

**Encourage** participants to ask questions and share their thoughts on applying SMART goals to their eating disorder recovery.

### Part Two

**Invite** group members to think about a goal they want to set to further their recovery this week. Ask them to write it down on "Setting SMART Goals" (Appendix 7A) using the following prompt:

> Think about a goal you want to set to further your recovery this week. Can you transform it into a SMART goal?

**Allocate** time for group members to utilize the handout in Appendix 7A, which will assist them in transforming their goals into SMART goals. This process may involve reevaluating their previous strategies and considering new approaches that align with the criteria of SMART goals.

**Encourage** group members to share their goals with the group.

**Facilitate** a discussion by asking, How did using the SMART goal format require you to approach goal-setting differently than in your previous experiences?

### Facilitators' Forum

Goal-setting can sometimes prompt anxiety or perfectionistic tendencies in individuals with eating disorders. Facilitators should be mindful of these potential triggers and prepared to offer support and reassurance as needed. Remind participants that progress is more important than perfection.

## Discussion 7.1 – Great Expectations

Many people begin their work in eating disorder recovery with unrealistic expectations of what the process entails or how long it takes. They may underestimate the challenges involved and subsequently experience frustration when their progress deviates from these initial expectations.

Recovery is not a linear process. It requires behavioral and psychological shifts. Understanding the complexities of the recovery process can help maintain the stamina needed to recover.

**Invite** group members to think back to when they started to address their eating disorder. It could be when they first noticed it was a problem and tried to make changes independently or when they first got help from professionals.

**Ask** the following prompt and allow group members to share their responses:

What was your understanding of what recovery or what being recovered meant when you first recognized your eating disorder as a problem? Can you recall thoughts or feelings you may have had regarding how long it may take to recover or how hard it would be?

Deepen the discussion by asking:

- What information or advice do you wish you had received when you first began eating disorder treatment? Why?
- Is there anything you wish your providers told your loved ones? If so, what and why?
- Do you have the skills to recover from your eating disorder? If not, what do you think you must learn or practice to make more progress in recovery?

### Facilitators' Forum

The absence of a universally agreed-upon definition of recovery means that group members may hold different conceptions of what it entails. When facilitators observe misaligned ideas about recovery among group members, it can create a sense of inaccessibility or the perception of doing recovery "wrong." In such instances, facilitators should emphasize recovery's nebulous nature and empower group members to define it on their terms. Facilitators are encouraged to support participants in envisioning a personal recovery that feels fulfilling and worth fighting for, recognizing that each individual's path may differ.

## Overcoming Experiential Avoidance

Experiential avoidance is the desire or attempt to avoid distressing and therefore unwanted internal experiences such as emotions, thoughts, memories, and bodily sensations. It refers to avoiding discomfort and seeking the safety and control of what is known, thereby providing short-term relief. Experiential avoidance can occur around body and food-specific internal experiences and distressing thoughts or core beliefs like "I'm worthless" or "I will never be good enough." Additionally, experiential avoidance often gives rise to feelings of anxiety, depression, and boredom.

Recovery from an eating disorder requires group members' willingness to take risks. In a group setting, this might look like members encouraging each other to face the challenges of trying new foods, eating in situations they have avoided, or abstaining from weighing themselves. For some, the process requires uncovering painful emotional experiences necessary for them to move through. As facilitators, it is essential to maintain a supportive and encouraging atmosphere, recognizing and celebrating each individual's progress no matter how small, keeping in mind recovery happens incrementally; every step toward recovery counts.

### Activity 7.3 – From Stuck to Empowered: Overcoming Challenges

Recovery requires a willingness to feel discomfort. It entails tolerating thoughts of potential failure or doubts about one's ability to recover. For participants to stay committed to eating disorder recovery, facilitators may encourage members to anchor themselves to their valued directions, such as their growing family or career aspirations. These anchors may serve as a guiding "north star" that helps make the short-term discomfort feel worthwhile. Throughout this process, individuals gradually learn that the distress they experience is bearable and temporary, and they emerge on the other side with newfound strength and resilience.

### Materials:

- Worksheet "From Stuck to Empowered: Overcoming Challenges" (Appendix 7B)
- For in-person groups, provide paper and writing utensils for group members.
- For virtual groups, members can gather their writing materials or utilize electronic devices for the activity.

**Begin** by introducing the concept of feeling stuck in recovery. Discuss what that means for group members by asking the following prompt and allowing them to share their responses:

> Think about a specific thought or behavior that keeps you stuck in your eating disorder or feel stagnant in your recovery.

**Use** the worksheet "From Stuck to Empowered: Overcoming Challenges" (Appendix 7B) and allow time for members to fill it out. This worksheet provides four columns: the problem or stuck point, what they have tried, the outcome, and what they could do differently.

**Invite** group members to share one row of the handout with the group (their stuck point or problem, what they have tried, the outcome, and what they could do differently).

**Further** the discussion to stimulate reflection by asking:

- How can you leverage your strengths and past successes in overcoming challenges to tackle this particular obstacle in your recovery?
- What support or assistance do you need to implement your ideas around what you can try differently? How can you access or cultivate that support system?
- How does overcoming this challenge align with your recovery goals and aspirations? How will it contribute to the life you want to live?
- Do you want accountability from the group when you meet next to help push through some of the discomforts?

### Facilitators' Forum

Invite participants to share examples of instances in their past where they have felt stuck while attempting to make changes, whether directly related to their eating disorder or not. This exercise encourages group members to delve into their personal experiences and explore strategies to break free from those stagnant situations. By reflecting on how they managed to get "unstuck," they can uncover valuable insights and lessons they may apply to their current eating disorder recovery.

## Discussion 7.2 – The Recovery Empowerment Plan

The primary focus of this activity is to assist group members in identifying obstacles that impede their progress in their eating disorder recovery and contribute to feeling stagnant. By sharing experiences and offering mutual support, participants can collaboratively develop actionable plans for change. This collective effort fosters a supportive community that can inspire group members to push past the obstacles keeping them stuck in their eating disorders.

**Introduce** the discussion, emphasizing that allowing group members to hold each other accountable can be a powerful way to follow through with the "doing" that recovery requires.

**Ask** the following prompt:

> Take a moment to reflect on obstacles you may be facing in your eating disorder recovery. Consider what things you still hold onto that represent your eating disorder, diet culture, or unattainable ideals or goals. These could be objects, beliefs, or behaviors. What are some of the hardest things to let go of and why?

**Explore** the impact of holding on to these items, thought patterns, or behaviors. Encourage them to reflect on why these items, thoughts, or behaviors have been challenging to abandon. Help participants recognize how holding on to them may hinder their progress in recovery by asking questions such as:

- How does holding on to this item, thought, or behavior impact your ability to recover from your eating disorder?
- Does this item, thought, or behavior symbolize a deeper struggle or issue? If so, what might that be?
- How can you address the underlying struggle or issue related to the item, thought, or behavior you identified?
- What may be the benefit(s) of letting this item, thought, or behavior go?

**Ask** group members if they feel ready to commit to letting go of one of their identified items, thoughts, or behaviors.

- For group members who identify a behavior or item, ask them to identify a first step they would commit to taking.
- For group members who identify a thought, ask them to describe how they would engage with this thought pattern differently (such as reframing).

**Consider** allocating time for participants to check in on their progress during future sessions or provide ongoing support and encouragement.

### Facilitators' Forum

For groups where enough members identify their scales as barriers to recovery, facilitators may consider following up this discussion with a scale smash, which can be empowering and cathartic. This activity involves participants destroying scales as a symbolic act of breaking free from the unhealthy grip of numbers and self-worth tied to weight. Physically smashing the scale can be a transformative experience, symbolizing the rejection of society's obsession with weight and embracing self-acceptance. It serves as a reminder that one's worth is not measured by a number but rather by unique qualities that make each individual whole.

## Fusion and Defusion

Steven Hays, the developer of ACT, coined the term "Cognitive Fusion."[4] It is the attachment to our thoughts to the extent we believe they are truths. It is important to note that thoughts in this case include internal experiences such as beliefs, assumptions, attitudes, and memories. When one experiences cognitive fusion, they are so "fused" with their thoughts that they cannot separate themselves from them. Instead, the thoughts become their reality.

In the following activities, we introduce the concepts of cognitive fusion and defusion. Opportunities are provided for group members to see themselves apart from eating disorder thoughts and practice the skill of cognitive defusion. Furthermore, the discussion delves into the factors that may influence the preference for defusion skills over CBT thought challenging approaches or DBT distress tolerance skills in specific situations.

### Discussion 7.3 – Exploring Cognitive Defusion Strategies

Cognitive fusion and cognitive defusion are especially salient concepts in eating disorder recovery because it is hard to separate one's thoughts from the entrenched eating disorder thoughts. The thoughts and associated feelings become an identity. The work of recovery requires separating the thoughts from the person. One effective technique for achieving this detachment is cognitive defusion, a process commonly employed in ACT.

### Materials:

• Handout "ACT Defusion Techniques" (Appendix 7C)

**Introduce** the concepts of cognitive fusion and cognitive defusion. Cognitive fusion is the experience of becoming so attached to our thoughts, so stuck in thinking patterns, that we become "fused" to them. When experiencing cognitive fusion, we cannot separate ourselves from our thoughts. Cognitive defusion is the process of noticing and observing thoughts and allowing thoughts to be recognized as just thoughts rather than commands or rules. This practice enables the thinker to notice the thoughts and decide which ones are workable, which ones to buy into, and which are proverbial junk mail.

**Explain** that relying solely on logic may not be effective when someone believes their eating disorder thoughts are true or when anxiety activates the threat system. In such situations, the prefrontal cortex, the part of the brain that allows one to access logic and reason, is "offline" as one's internal alarm system is in fight/flight/freeze mode. It is in those situations when thought defusion techniques can be valuable.

**Direct** the group's attention to the handout "ACT Defusion Techniques" (Appendix 7C). Encourage participants to review the various defusion techniques listed.

**Facilitate** a discussion by asking:

• Have you used any of these techniques before? Can you envision yourself using them in the future?
• What potential barriers might hinder you from trying one of these techniques?
• How can you overcome these barriers?

*Facilitators' Forum*

As facilitators, it is essential to acknowledge the challenges participants face when attempting to break free from the grip of their eating disorder thought patterns. Being fused with these thoughts can create a sense of being trapped and may impede progress toward recovery. Participants may rely on logic or what is commonly known as "the healthy voice" to counteract the influence of the eating disorder voice. While this approach may be helpful when challenging certain disordered thoughts, it can sometimes lead to a draining back-and-forth battle with the eating disorder voice, tirelessly vying for control. These are the times when these cognitive defusion techniques are especially useful.

## Activity 7.4 – Making It Funny

This exercise provides an opportunity for group members to practice cognitive defusion techniques. It requires members to use the mindfulness skills of noticing and observing along with humor to build emotional resilience.

## Materials:

- For in-person groups, provide paper and writing utensils for group members.
- For virtual groups, members can gather their writing materials or utilize electronic devices for the activity.

**Ask** the prompt:

> Write down some of your eating disorder thoughts that pop up repeatedly.
> Practice cognitive defusion by writing the thoughts as "I notice I have a thought that _____."

**Provide** an example to illustrate the process. For instance, you might share the thought, "I notice I have the thought that pizza is scary."

**Invite** group members to share their thoughts using the format "I noticed I have the thought _____."

**Prompt** further discussion by asking questions:

- What happens if you go along with this thought? How does it influence your behavior?
- Is this thought workable? Specifically, will it get you closer to recovery or keep you stuck in the eating disorder?

**Transition** to the humor aspect of the exercise. Guide group members in finding ways to approach their thoughts with less seriousness. Encourage them to explore humorous perspectives by asking questions such as, *How can this thought be funny? Can you try saying it in a funny voice? Can you come up with a hilarious visual representation?* For instance, using the example of pizza being scary, an amusing visual representation could involve imagining a pizza with fangs chasing you.

**Reflect** on the exercise as a group by asking:

- How does engaging in comical cognitive defusion alter your perception of this thought?
- In what ways does this approach open up new possibilities for change that you may not have considered before?
- Can you envision applying this skill and other cognitive defusion techniques to additional recurring eating disorder thoughts? Explain.

### Facilitators' Forum

Some ways to enhance this activity may include:

- Give group members humorous prompts or questions to stimulate their creativity and help them approach their thoughts with humor. For example, ask them to imagine their eating disorder thought as a character in a comedy sketch or devise a funny tagline related to their thought.
- Encourage group members to express their thoughts creatively by drawing, writing short humorous stories, or creating funny captions for images. An experiential approach allows individual expression and can lead to unique insights and perspectives.

## Unpacking the Emotional Burden: Guilt and Shame in Eating Disorders

Guilt commonly arises in individuals with eating disorders during the recovery process when they resist engaging in their symptoms. They may experience guilt when they opt for a meal that is not the lowest in calories on the menu or consume both halves of a sandwich. For individuals dealing with compulsive exercise, guilt often arises when they cut a workout short, skip it to enjoy dinner with friends, or take a rest day due to illness.

Guilt often leads to shame and self-loathing, which can feel physically intolerable and inescapable. To quiet this guilt, one may engage in compensatory eating disorder behaviors; for example, restricting, purging by self-induced vomiting, or increasing the duration or intensity of exercise. While or after engaging in these behaviors, one may feel guilty or ashamed for keeping the behavior a secret or for "choosing" their eating disorder over spending time with friends and family. These efforts may eventually backfire as deprivation, be it actual deprivation via food restriction or mental deprivation by labeling certain foods as "bad" or forbidden, more often than not leads to bingeing or feeling out of control around food. Although it is a response to compensatory behaviors, they are left feeling guilty yet again. This pattern is why eating disorder behaviors are often depicted in a cycle; the cycle of one compensatory behavior follows another. Thus the cycle of guilt continues.

Shame is the belief that one is inherently wrong or inadequate. Shame is the internalized guilt that someone feels. Guilt from feeling bad for engaging in behavior one sees as bad, combined with shame, leads to the maintenance of eating disorder behaviors.

### Discussion 7.4 – Transforming Guilt and Shame into Empowerment

This discussion will help group members to practice vulnerability by identifying aspects of their eating disorder that have caused them to feel guilty or ashamed. Recognizing that others share these thoughts and fears can help them see the common humanity in their struggles. This realization is key to developing self-compassion and reducing feelings of shame.

**Ask** group members the following prompt.

> How has your eating disorder hindered you from living a life aligned with your core values?

For instance, did they miss out on time with family or friends that was important to them? Did a preoccupation with food or their bodies keep them from engaging in or enjoying certain experiences to the fullest (i.e., vacations, study abroad, new job, etc.)?

**Invite** members to share how their eating disorder kept them from living a life aligned with their values.

Further the discussion by asking:

- What aspects of your eating disorder or recovery trigger feelings of guilt or shame?
- How does guilt or shame keep you stuck in your eating disorder?
- What has helped to reduce guilt or shame in your recovery?
- How can guilt and the associated regret be helpful in recovery?

- How can you navigate the process of grieving the losses and precious moments missed due to the eating disorder while finding ways to honor and cherish those experiences in your present and future?
- How can you cultivate self-compassion and understanding, recognizing that the eating disorder was an attempt to care for yourself when you lacked alternative coping mechanisms or strategies?

### Facilitators' Forum

When addressing the themes of guilt or shame in a group setting, facilitators should emphasize that exploring these topics is not to amplify their already challenging emotions. Instead, the aim is to utilize these uncomfortable, sad, or regretful emotions as a catalyst for a more profound examination of one's experience with the eating disorder. By delving into these feelings, group members can gain insight into their emotions within the context of their disorder, ultimately leading to personal growth and healing.

To conclude the group session, setting aside time for the collective release of guilt or shame can be valuable. This release can be facilitated through a communal breath exercise, guiding participants to take deep, intentional breaths together. Alternatively, encouraging participants to engage in a self-hug can provide a comforting gesture that promotes self-compassion and self-care. By embracing themselves with a gentle and nurturing touch, participants can symbolically embrace their vulnerabilities and acknowledge their need for kindness and understanding.

## Activity 7.5 – Rules Were Made to Be Broken

In this activity, participants are asked to identify and question their rules and assumptions regarding food, exercise, weight, and body shape and size. By engaging in open and reflective discussions, group members can explore the origins of these rules and assess whether they help or harm them.

Through this process, group members can recognize that these rules often contribute to feelings of guilt and shame. By challenging and questioning these beliefs, participants can begin to cultivate self-compassion and free themselves from the constraints these rules impose.

As the group collectively examines these rules, they may discover they were adopted to manage emotions and protect themselves from potential rejection. By gaining awareness of the underlying motivations behind these rules, participants can develop healthier coping mechanisms and a more positive relationship with their bodies and food. Ultimately, this activity aims to support participants in embracing freedom from self-imposed restrictions, fostering self-compassion, and promoting a more authentic and fulfilling life aligned with their true values.

## Materials:

- Worksheet "Food Rules" (Appendix 7D)
- For in-person groups, provide writing utensils for group members.
- For virtual groups, members can gather their writing materials or utilize electronic devices for the activity.

**Distribute** the worksheet "Food Rules" (Appendix 7D). For virtual groups, the worksheet can be displayed using a screen-sharing feature.

**Introduce** the prompt:

> Consider a specific food rule that keeps you stuck in your eating disorder.

**Allot** time for members to fill out the worksheet.
**Ask:**

- Where did your rule come from?
- Did you feel that your rule strongly related to one of the four influencing factors on the worksheet? If so, which one?
- How does looking at your food rule through the lens of one of these four factors help to understand your difficulty in rejecting this rule? Does this perspective reduce your guilt or shame?
- Why are you afraid of breaking this rule? What emotions would you experience if you pushed yourself to break this rule?
- What would be the consequence of keeping this rule? What are the benefits of breaking this rule?

### Facilitators' Forum

Regarding rules that deal with food or nutrition, group members might *know* on a basic level that their food rule is irrational or scientifically inaccurate, but sometimes still find it hard to truly believe it. In a climate where nutrition misinformation is so pervasive and accessible, especially on social media, it is not surprising that false information gets easily reinforced. The dietitian can assess whether providing more nutrition information would be helpful.

## Cultivating Self-Compassion in Eating Disorder Recovery

Self-compassion is turning compassion inward by showing yourself kindness. Numerous studies have shown self-compassion to be a protective factor against poor body image, disordered eating, and eating disorders.[5] Although the eating disorder is a coping skill and often provides immediate comfort, the eating disorder voice can be critical and sound cruel. Using self-compassion allows members to reframe this harsh self-talk and transform this language into a softer, kinder inner dialogue.

There is also a physiological benefit to self-compassion work in eating disorder recovery. Self-compassion can activate our parasympathetic nervous system, also called the "rest and digest" state, which can help relax the body. In contrast, self-criticism activates the threat system, triggering the "fight or flight" response and heightening emotional distress. This sustained distress reinforces the disorder, creating a sense of being trapped and impeding progress.

## Activity 7.6 – Connecting with Compassion: The Self-Compassionate Letter Writing Experience

For this activity, inspired by the self-compassionate letter-writing exercise developed by Dr. Kristin Neff, group members are encouraged to connect with their self-compassionate voice by writing a heartfelt letter to themselves.[6] This exercise focuses on fostering self-compassion, specifically in the context of eating disorder recovery. By engaging in this process, participants will have the opportunity to offer themselves understanding, kindness, and support while acknowledging the challenges they have faced and the progress they have made. This activity aims to nurture self-compassion and explore its positive impact on their recovery. Participants will also be encouraged to notice the physical sensations and emotional experiences associated with engaging in self-compassion.

## Materials:

- For in-person groups, provide paper and writing utensils for group members.
- For virtual groups, members can gather writing materials or utilize electronic devices.

**Begin** by asking group members to reflect on their eating disorder recovery and a specific moment when they encountered challenges or setbacks. Allow them a few moments to bring this situation to mind.

**Guide** the group by asking them to think about the following prompts:

1. What was the challenging moment you encountered in your eating disorder recovery?
2. How did you feel during that time?
3. What thoughts or emotions arose as a result?
4. Reflect on the progress you have made since that challenging moment.

Allow for a pause.

Next, provide the following instruction:

> Think of that challenging moment in your eating disorder recovery. Write a letter to yourself using a self-compassionate tone and approach. As you write, offer understanding, kindness, and support to yourself. Acknowledge the difficulties you faced and express compassion for the emotions you experienced. Emphasize self-acceptance, encouragement, and reassurance. Treat yourself with the same care and compassion you would extend to a dear friend going through a similar struggle.

**Invite** group members to write a letter to themselves using their self-compassionate voice. Remember, this is compassion turned inwards and directed at themselves, so this voice is understanding, kind, and gentle.

**Allow** members to share their letters with the group aloud if they would like.

**Facilitate** a group discussion by posing the following questions:

- How did engaging with yourself compassionately in the context of your eating disorder recovery feel?
- Did you notice any physical sensations or emotional shifts while writing the letter? If so, what?
- What was it like to hear the letters of other group members?
- Can you identify anyone in your support network who can help you access and cultivate your compassionate voice? If so, how would their words sound?
- What strategies or practices can make it easier for you to engage with yourself compassionately on a regular basis throughout your eating disorder recovery?

### Facilitators' Forum

If group members struggle to tap into their self-compassionate voice, they may find it helpful to imagine their treatment team responding to them in a supportive and reassuring manner. Drawing upon the compassionate perspectives of their trusted team can serve as a starting point for accessing self-compassion. They can also consider the supportive words and guidance they would receive from a dependable person in their life, such as a parent, spouse, close friend, or mentor. By envisioning these sources of support and compassion, group members can begin to cultivate self-compassion and provide themselves with the understanding and kindness they deserve.

Facilitators may find it useful to differentiate self-compassion from self-pity or going too easy on oneself. Cultivating the ability to turn inward and practice compassion toward oneself allows one to see their struggles while also taking ownership of past struggles or mistakes. This growth-oriented mindset can be a key tool to challenge thoughts of regret or shame for struggling with an eating disorder.

### Exploring the Link Between Perfectionism and Eating Disorders

Perfectionism is widely recognized as a risk factor and a key element in maintaining eating disorders. Extensive research indicates that perfectionism hinders successful treatment outcomes for individuals coping with eating disorders and those with anxiety and depressive disorders.[7] The goals of treatment interventions that target perfectionism include decreasing rigid thinking and behavior while increasing flexibility. Working toward finding "comfort in the gray" instead of seeking safety and control "in the black and white" is critical in treating eating disorders.

It is essential to point out that giving up perfectionism does not mean one no longer strives to meet goals. It does not mean that someone is "giving up" or "does not care" anymore. It is about identifying areas where unrelenting standards do not serve them. In most cases, these standards maintain core beliefs related to inadequacy and that worth is determined by what they do or look like instead of who they are.

### Discussion 7.5 – Breaking Free: Recovering from Perfectionism

In this discussion, participants will be encouraged to explore the relationship between their eating disorders and perfectionism. Recognizing and challenging unrealistic expectations is a crucial aspect of eating disorder recovery. As part of this process, group members will engage in self-reflection to acknowledge the futility of perfectionism and cultivate a greater acceptance of imperfection as a necessary step toward healing.

**Ask** the prompt:

> To recover from an eating disorder, you must recover from perfectionism. What does that mean to you? Do you agree?

**Allow** group members to share their responses.
**Further** the discussion by asking:

- What feelings arise when you hear the idea of recovering from perfectionism?
- Consider how perfectionism interacts with your eating disorder. How and where does it appear (in the group, eating, body image, recovery, relationships)? What reinforces it?
- What are the benefits of letting go of perfectionism?

- What are the challenges and drawbacks associated with being perfectionistic?
- How does perfectionism hinder your ability to fully engage with the world?
- Why do you think many people with eating disorders identify as perfectionists?

### Facilitators' Forum

Perfectionism is a complex topic that intersects with various aspects of our lives, including diet culture, where it can be deeply ingrained. Diet culture promotes achieving a perfect diet, following a singular "right" way of eating or exercising, and exerting control over one's weight. These expectations perpetuate perfectionistic tendencies. Moreover, perfectionism is linked to symptoms and behaviors such as bingeing, purging, avoidance, and procrastination.

To further explore the connection between perfectionism and diet culture, consider asking group members how they observe perfectionism manifesting in diet culture. This discussion can open up new avenues for exploration and understanding. For more insights on diet culture, refer to Chapter 8.

## Discussion 7.6 – What If I Fail?

In the pursuit of perfection, participants may avoid situations that may lead to perceived "failures" or setbacks. However, by doing so, they miss out on valuable learning and personal growth opportunities. In this discussion, group members are encouraged to reflect on a specific instance when they didn't meet their goals or fell short in some way. Participants will explore strategies for approaching their inner critic through the lens of self-compassion. By adopting a self-compassionate approach, participants can reduce feelings of shame or guilt associated with mistakes or "failures" and enhance their cognitive flexibility.

**Introduce** the prompt:

Recall a specific instance when you experienced a sense of failure or received feedback that suggested you had failed at something.

Can you identify the messages your inner critic conveyed during that time?

**Allow** time to reflect on what that perceived failure meant to them. Encourage them to consider how those messages made them feel emotionally and physically.

**Invite** group members to share their memories and reflections with the group.

**Facilitate** a group discussion by asking how it feels to hear a group member's inner critic and what a compassionate response to the critic might be.

**Ask** each group member to practice giving themselves compassion aloud. Facilitators may model this language if the group has difficulty accessing their self-compassionate voice.

**Reflect** on the exercise by posing questions to the group:

- How does it feel to give yourself compassion as opposed to criticism?
- What is the difference between constructive feedback and self-criticism?
- What are the barriers to providing yourself with compassion? (i.e., the idea self-criticism can motivate, toughen you up, and push you to do better while being compassionate will make you lazy, is an excuse for failing).
- How does fear of judgment from others reinforce the inner critic and serve as a barrier to taking risks, thereby preventing growth?

### Facilitators' Forum

Perfectionism impedes creativity by preventing people from taking risks that may lead to needed growth. Still thinking about their memory, invite the group to contemplate the idea that "failure is feedback." Through this lens, what was the learning, or the gift, of the "failure"?

## Notes

1 Rie, S. M. de la, G. Noordenbos, and van Furth E. F. 2005. "Quality of Life and Eating Disorders." *Quality of Life Research* 14 (6): 1511–1521. https://doi.org/10.1007/s11136-005-0585-0.

2 Juarascio, Adrienne, Jena Shaw, Evan M. Forman, C. Alix Timko, James D. Herbert, Meghan L. Butryn, and Michael Lowe. 2013. "Acceptance and Commitment Therapy for Eating Disorders: Clinical Applications of a Group Treatment." *Journal of Contextual Behavioral Science* 2 (3–4): 85–94. https://doi.org/10.1016/j.jcbs.2013.08.001.

3 Doran, George T. 1981. "There's a SMART Way to Write Management's Goals and Objectives." *Management Review* 70 (11): 35–36.

4 Hayes, Steven C., Kirk Strosahl, and Kelly G. Wilson. 2012. "Chapter 3, Psychological Flexibility as a Unified Model of Human Functioning." In *Acceptance and Commitment Therapy the Process and Practice of Mindful Change*. New York: Guilford Press.

5 Braun, Tosca D., Crystal L. Park, and Amy Gorin. 2016. "Self-Compassion, Body Image, and Disordered Eating: A Review of the Literature." *Body Image* 17: 117–131. https://doi.org/10.1016/j.bodyim.2016.03.003.

6 Neff, Kristen. 2015. "Exercise 3: Exploring Self-Compassion through Writing." *Self*, June 10, 2015. https://self-compassion.org/exercise-3-exploring-self-compassion-writing/.

7 Levinson, Cheri A., Leigh C. Brosof, Irina A. Vanzhula, Laura Bumberry, Stephanie Zerwas, and Cynthia M. Bulik. 2017. "Perfectionism Group Treatment for Eating Disorders in an Inpatient, Partial Hospitalization, and Outpatient Setting." *European Eating Disorders Review* 25 (6): 579–585. https://doi.org/10.1002/erv.2557.

# Appendix 7A – Setting SMART Goals (for Activity 7.2)

**Goal Idea:**

Is my goal:

- **Specific**: The goal should be clear, well-defined, and unambiguous.

  Example: Eating a breakfast that follows my meal plan for 7 days.

- **Measurable:** The goal must include criteria to allow you to track your progress and know when you achieve it.

  Example: Keeping a food log for a full 7 days.

- **Achievable:** The goal must be realistic and feel possible.

  Example: Not weighing myself more than once this week.

- **Relevant:** The goal needs to be related to a larger goal, which in our case is recovery from the eating disorder.

  Example: I will attend my work's lunch and learn this week.

- **Time-Limited**: The goal must have a time limit to keep one focused to avoid avoiding.

  Example: I will not weigh myself for the next 7 days.

**SMART Goal** (rewrite of goal idea):

# Appendix 7B – From Stuck to Empowered: Overcoming Challenges (for Activity 7.3)

| Stuck Point/ Problem | What Has Been Tried | Outcome | What Could Be Done Differently? |
|---|---|---|---|
| *Example: Skipping breakfast* | *Setting breakfast out the night before*<br>*Making a plan for breakfasts for the week* | *Not looking at the plan*<br>*Forgetting to put breakfast out* | *Texting friend a picture of breakfast set out for 1 week*<br>*Texting dietitian after eating breakfast for 1 week* |
| | | | |
| | | | |
| | | | |
| | | | |

# Appendix 7C – Defusion Techniques (for Discussion 7.3)

## ACT Defusion Techniques

*Just Noticing:* Say to yourself, "I notice I'm having a thought that/of . . ." To take it a step further, you can label the thought, which may be an inner experience. For example, "I am noticing I am having the thought that I am inadequate." Additionally, you can label the thinking error (cognitive distortion, to use the language of CBT). For example, "I am noticing my mind is over-generalizing again."

*Thank You Mind:* Although it sounds silly, practicing noticing a thought and expressing gratitude to your mind can help you detach from the thought. In most cases, our mind is simply trying to protect us, albeit in a way that is ultimately harmful. Some find it helpful to add a hand gesture to indicate, "I got you, but I got this one," and even a little sarcasm, as our minds can be reactive and exaggerate threats. An example is "Thanks, mind, for looking out for me, but I'm all good," or whatever works to help you stop being bullied by your thoughts and taking all of them so seriously.

*Simply Observing:* Watching your thoughts without judgment and instead with curiosity and openness can allow you to let the thoughts come and go. The idea here is not to try to control or change your thoughts. For instance, you may be ordering food at a restaurant for dinner and notice the thought that you should not be eating out again since you ordered in at work. (This breaks your eating disorder rule). Simply noticing this thought would mean you don't try to make it go away, judge, or challenge it. Instead, you notice it, return to the present, and order dinner. If it comes back, you can simply observe it again and shift your focus back to the present moment.

*Make It Funny:* It's hard to take thoughts seriously if you are saying them in the voice of a cartoon character. You can add a layer to the absurdity by visualizing a cartoon character saying them. In this vein, saying them over and over can help you see how ridiculous they are.

For instance, "Pizza is scary" when said multiple times in a funny voice with a visual of pizza chasing you makes it hard to take that thought seriously. Repeating the thoughts can take the meaning away from them; all you are left with are sounds.

# Appendix 7D – Food Rules (Activity 7.5)

| Food Rule: | |
|---|---|
| Consider whether these factors influence the difficulty in letting go of this rule. In the column on the right, make any pertinent notes to contribute to the discussion. | |
| **Emotional Attachment:**<br>Food and eating habits can be deeply ingrained in one's personal and cultural identity. Letting go of long-held beliefs and practices can be challenging, even when presented with contradictory evidence. | |
| **Cognitive Biases:**<br>Human beings are prone to cognitive biases, such as confirmation bias, which leads individuals to seek out information that confirms their pre-existing beliefs while ignoring or dismissing conflicting information. This bias makes it difficult to accept new information that challenges their existing beliefs about nutrition. | |
| **Influence of Social Networks:**<br>In today's digital age, social media plays a significant role in shaping people's opinions and behaviors. Misinformation about nutrition spreads rapidly through social networks, creating echo chambers reinforcing false beliefs. This collective reinforcement makes it harder for individuals to break away from their misguided notions. | |
| **Scientific Literacy:**<br>Understanding complex scientific concepts related to nutrition can be challenging for the general population. Misinterpretation or misrepresentation of scientific studies can further contribute to confusion and the perpetuation of false beliefs. | |

# Chapter 8

# Liberation from Diet Culture

## Using a Social Justice Lens in Eating Disorder Recovery

The messages internalized about health and bodies from mainstream culture, marketing, and social media exert a powerful influence that overwhelmingly promotes the "thin ideal" and pressures individuals to conform to unrealistic beauty standards. This chapter aims to deconstruct those messages, exploring the entities that profit from body (and health) insecurity and methods to cultivate body neutrality and, eventually, appreciation.

To cultivate a healthy relationship with one's body and food, examining the underlying factors contributing to and sustaining body insecurity, shame, and anxiety surrounding food is vital. Often group members will recall schoolyard jabs made about the size of their belly or thighs, their mothers putting them on diets, or their doctor who told them they needed to cut down on "junk food" because they were bigger than they "should" be. While negative comments certainly play a role, it is crucial to go beyond individual experiences and acknowledge the larger societal factors embedded in Western culture that contribute to the formation and perpetuation of harmful beliefs surrounding food and its relationship with our bodies.

A sociocultural perspective is embraced throughout this chapter due to the profound influence it has on individuals' mental health. This perspective emphasizes how larger cultural systems impact individuals' thoughts, behaviors, and relationships with food and their bodies. By acknowledging this sociocultural context, we can better understand and address the complex dynamics of social justice and diet culture within the group therapy setting.

Drawing from a range of therapeutic modalities and approaches, including Solution-Focused Therapy (SFT), Cognitive Behavioral Therapy (CBT), Acceptance and Commitment Therapy (ACT), Positive Psychology, Interpersonal Therapy, Psychoeducation, Narrative Therapy, media literacy, and advocacy, we will explore their practical applications in addressing the harmful influences of diet culture, promoting body acceptance, and empowering individuals in their recovery process.

In addition to these therapeutic approaches, this chapter embraces a feminist perspective. This perspective recognizes the systemic nature of oppression and

DOI: 10.4324/9781003430964-11

emphasizes dismantling patriarchal structures that contribute to body shaming, objectification, and unrealistic beauty standards. By adopting a feminist lens, the group facilitators create a safe and inclusive space where individuals can explore the intersectionality of their identities and how these converge with their experiences of body image and disordered eating. This approach promotes critical consciousness, challenges dominant cultural narratives, and supports group members in reclaiming autonomy over their bodies while fostering collective action for social change.

## The Diet Culture Landscape

Registered Dietitian and prominent author Christy Harrison describes diet culture as "a system of beliefs that worships thinness and equates it to health and moral virtue."[1] Harrison explains that central to diet culture is the idea that thinness can further a person's social standing and that there is a correct way to eat. Through this demonization and promotion of certain foods and a deeply flawed, weight-centric idea of health, people who do not fit this narrow standard of "health" are mistreated.[2]

Diet culture perpetuates eating disorders in many ways, preventing people from trusting their instincts around their bodies and choices. Reimagining one's body as something to be trusted requires education about this learned system that commandeered that body trust in the first place. Learning that the "thin ideal," food trends, and some dietary recommendations are socially constructed and motivated by profit and consumerism is empowering. It allows members to more readily reject messaging that there is one right way to eat and that their body is the problem. The group can work together to foster personal and communal growth by acknowledging and addressing societal constructs and hierarchies.

This zoomed-out view allows group members to soften their anger at the harmful, formative messages and the people who reinforced them over their lifetime. It also allows group members to find a space of compassion for themselves. How could individuals not feel ashamed of their bodies or food choices when diet culture's job was to create a feeling of inadequacy? The aim is for them to arrive at a place of understanding that others were duped as well. The diet culture rollercoaster, which has instilled in individuals the belief that their bodies must change to be considered acceptable and attractive, can only be confronted when the blame is removed from themselves and those around them. Everyone has been affected by diet culture's toxic messages; everyone has been a victim.

The benefits of group activities and discussions centered around diet culture and social justice include decreasing shame while increasing self-compassion and empowerment. Group members will have encountered differences in their lived experiences in diet culture and conforming to relatively homogeneous beauty standards, but they are all impacted. Diet and beauty messages are everywhere. We often say in our group, "It's no wonder you feel this way! Just think about how often you hear 'such-and-such' message." If group members can stop blaming themselves for feeling compelled to conform to these appearance standards, an opening is created for self-compassion.

While group members are encouraged to advocate for dismantling unhealthy messages about food and bodies, it is important to acknowledge the vast scale of these issues and the challenges involved in finding solutions. The focus should remain on individuals working toward eating disorder recovery, which can be conceptualized as powerful acts of resistance against these harmful messages. Each person has the potential to become a proverbial lighthouse, guiding others toward healing. By strengthening their skills and reducing the influence of diet culture on themselves, group members can create a ripple effect that positively impacts the healing process of others.

### The "Thin Ideal"

Body image experts use the term "thin ideal" to describe this narrow standard of beauty.[3] Clinical psychologist Niva Piran suggests that "embodying this ideal" is a more precise way of describing the act of conforming to the "thin ideal," as this standard encompasses numerous privileges linked to factors such as weight, body type, age, race, ethnicity, gender identity, and social status.[4],[5] We see this ideal everywhere. Cultural institutions such as mass media, beauty, and diet industries disseminate these messages regarding physical appearance as facts. While there is some variation in beauty standards across different cultures and individuals, certain beauty ideals are more pervasive and influential in mainstream culture than others. One of these ideals is the "thin ideal," which refers to the cultural preference for a slender or lean body type.

Unattainable beauty standards, including the "thin ideal," lead to pervasive body dissatisfaction and body comparison, setting the stage for developing an obsession with procuring the body that one cannot have without doing unnatural things to achieve it. When one's body does not measure up to the celebrated thin norm, the propensity for trying to fix the body becomes a compulsion.

A difficult truth that many who struggle with eating disorders must contend with at some point is that the pursuit of thinness perpetuates weight stigma. In other words, by restricting, purging, over-exercising, and using surgical interventions to force one's body to be a certain size, that person perpetuates the power that the "thin ideal" has as the favored, desirable body type.

## The Social Justice Intersection

A culture that sends and reinforces the message that one's value is determined by the size or shape of one's body or food choices normalizes and condones discrimination. By its very nature, a preoccupation with maintaining a certain physical appearance vilifies bodies outside this ideal. While there is no simple way to detach from the belief that self-worth is influenced by adherence to "healthy" eating or having a thin body, shifting thought patterns, implementing behavioral interventions, and acknowledging this as a social justice issue rather than simply a personal battle can catalyze change in eating disorder recovery.

The group provides a space for group members to acknowledge the challenges of living in a society that values certain body types and subjugates others based on weight and food choices. Members who have experienced marginalization due to ableism, weight stigma, or racism can share their experiences and educate the group about how these experiences have impacted their illness and recovery.

The group discussions and activities encourage group members to reflect on their privilege, including white privilege, thin privilege, cis privilege, straight/ heterosexual privilege, and economic privilege, and how such privilege has impacted their illness and recovery. Additionally, they examine how the widespread societal bias against fat bodies, known colloquially as "fatphobia," perpetuates thin privilege and contributes to the persistence of eating disorders.

Through these collective conversations, members gain a greater understanding of the systemic issues surrounding body image and eating disorders. This increased awareness empowers individuals to challenge societal norms, promote inclusivity, and work toward creating a more equitable and accepting society.

## Discussion 8.1 – The Social Justice Intersection

The purpose of this discussion is to explore the intricate relationship between body image, weight stigma, discrimination, and the broader concept of social justice. The objective is to provide a safe and inclusive space where group members can openly explore these topics and engage in meaningful conversations that promote reflection, empathy, and empowerment.

Facilitators will encourage personal reflection, inviting participants to delve into their own experiences with societal beauty standards, weight stigma, and discrimination. Examining these experiences allows members to deepen their understanding of their impact on individuals' self-perception and motivation to change.

Additionally, the concept of privilege is explored. Through this exploration, members are asked to consider how different forms of privilege intersect with issues related to body image and eating disorders, further expanding their understanding of the systemic biases that perpetuate these issues.

**Provide** a brief overview of the session's goals: to explore societal influences on body image, weight stigma, and discrimination and to discuss how these issues intersect with social justice.

### Part One – Personal Reflection

**Ask** group members to take a few moments to reflect on their experiences with societal beauty standards, body image, weight stigma, or discrimination.

Use prompts to guide their reflection:

Have you experienced weight stigma or discrimination due to your body size or food choices?

How has society's emphasis on thinness or specific body ideals influenced your self-worth or self-perception?

In what ways have societal beauty standards affected your relationship with food and your body?

Facilitate discussion, asking group members to share their reflections and personal experiences related to the prompts. Highlight the diverse experiences within the group and acknowledge the impact of societal influences on group members' sense of Self.

### Part Two – Privilege Reflection

Introduce the concept of privilege and its relevance to the topic.

Invite participants to reflect on the various types of privilege they may hold, such as white privilege, thin privilege, cis privilege, straight/heterosexual privilege, and economic privilege. Invite them to consider how these privileges may have affected their experiences with body image, weight stigma, and access to healthcare or resources related to their eating disorder.

Explore intersectionality by initiating a group discussion on intersectionality, emphasizing how different forms of privilege and marginalization merge and interact with each other. Encourage participants to share their reflections on how their privileges and experiences of marginalization have influenced their illness and recovery within the context of societal biases and discrimination (i.e., access to healthcare, comfort level seeking medical care, access to a variety of foods, or ability to go clothes shopping at a store).

Summarize the main insights and themes discussed during the session. If desired, provide resources, such as recommended readings or websites, for further exploration of the topic.

### Facilitators' Forum

A commitment to ongoing education and personal growth is vital to be effective facilitators. This commitment is especially significant in understanding and addressing social justice issues, intersectionality, and body image concerns. By staying informed about current research, emerging perspectives, and inclusive practices, facilitators can significantly enhance their ability to support group members. Embracing lifelong learning and being open to new ideas and approaches fosters an environment where facilitators can adapt to the ever-evolving societal landscape and create a safe space for diverse perspectives.

Staying abreast of social justice issues is imperative for facilitators. This involves understanding systemic oppression, discrimination, and privilege. Incorporating an intersectional approach in eating disorder treatment and eating disorder recovery means recognizing these diverse experiences and tailoring support to meet the unique needs of individuals from different backgrounds. It involves addressing the multiple layers of oppression and privilege that can affect their recovery and promoting more accepting, empathetic, and culturally competent care.

## The Business of Beauty

A quick look at social media trends, advertising campaigns, and influencers reflects a predominant image of what Western society considers to be a beautiful woman. This beauty ideal, rooted in colonialism and racism, idealizes European features. This standard dictates that a woman must be slim, toned, young, and voluptuous, with all body hair meticulously groomed or removed. Her skin should be white or light, and her hair should be long, straight, and perfectly styled. Additionally, she should wear trendy, fashionable clothing and accessories.[6,7]

The beauty industry is a fundamental part of discussions around beauty standards. In her 2022 book *Decolonizing Wellness*, Registered Dietitian Dalia Kinsey poignantly writes, "The beauty standard is elusive by design. It is meant to generate a sense of deficit and inadequacy in us so we will be motivated to buy more products that promise to fix us."[8] There is inherent manipulation when the industry that establishes beauty standards is also capitalizing on the sales of products that people believe will bring them confidence, satisfaction, and happiness.

When conducting groups about beauty standards, group facilitators should remind members that someone is profiting from their buy-in to these norms, and heavily at that. Beauty is big business. Industry sees advertising money as well-spent when consumers continue buying products perpetuating current beauty norms. This industry will remain too powerful until people can redefine beauty from the inside out instead of the outside in. People can only begin to rely more on products and things to *feel* beautiful once they recognize the beauty that is inherent within them.

In conversations about beauty standards, it is crucial to acknowledge that the existing trends are often impossible or difficult for many people to meet. For example, the trend of having large buttocks and a tiny waist, as popularized by celebrities, may be easier for some people to obtain due to their genetics. In contrast, others may turn to surgery or extreme diet and exercise regimens to obtain this. Similarly, increases in breast size, often considered desirable in Western culture, can be influenced by factors such as hormones, pregnancy, and weight fluctuations and may not be easily controlled.

It is important to remember that these trends are not universal or fixed; they can change rapidly and unpredictably. Attempting to meet certain standards or expectations constantly can be exhausting, stressful, and ultimately futile. Moreover, it can contribute to negative body image, eating disorders, and other mental and physical health issues.

### The Broad Conceptualization of Beauty

While the internalization of the "thin ideal" is a strong predictor of body image disturbances and eating disorders, the good news is that it is possible to ignore or resist conforming to this beauty standard.[9] Several separate research groups interviewed adolescent and adult females with a positive body image or who scored well on body esteem assessments. Through these interviews, a recurring theme surfaced. Beauty can be perceived more inclusively and expansively. Individuals with a positive body image typically had a broad perspective on physical beauty, recognizing that attractiveness can come in many forms, whether determined by mostly unchangeable factors such as body shape and weight or more flexible ones like fashion choices and hairstyles. Additionally, they emphasized positive internal qualities, such as self-confidence and self-acceptance, which played a crucial role in shaping the perception of beauty, not just in others but also in themselves, that is not aligned with socio-cultural beauty ideals.[10]

Individuals who had a more expansive perception of beauty tended to exhibit greater levels of body appreciation and self-compassion while also displaying lower levels of anti-fat attitudes, body surveillance, thin-ideal internalization, acceptance of cosmetic surgery, and social comparison related to body image, exercise, and eating.[11]

As described in Chapter 4, one benefit of the group format is that the community gets to know one another quite well and has the potential to redefine the way they think of beauty through how they see each other. In other words, when we take the time to truly know someone, we open ourselves up to discovering their beauty. Seeing others as beautiful through getting to know them and appreciating the person they are with all of their quirks, personality traits, and characteristics challenges the belief that someone's appearance conforming to a narrow definition of attractiveness is what makes them most beautiful. When the group works together to dismantle this narrow conceptualization of beauty, it allows members to gain new perspectives on how others perceive them and may enable them to see themselves in a new light.

## Discussion 8.2 – The Last Time I Felt Beautiful

This exercise can help group members recognize that beauty and self-worth are not solely dependent on external appearance but can also stem from personal qualities or experiences. It allows members to reflect on positive aspects of themselves that may not be related to their physical appearance, which can help promote self-acceptance and positive body image.

Society dictates what is on-trend, fashionable, and beautiful. This influence extends beyond material possessions and encompasses ideals surrounding bodies as well. The notion that body shapes and sizes can be altered to conform to ever-changing trends, akin to designer items, is a fallacy. This activity tasks group members to identify a time when they felt beautiful and discern between the beauty that felt unique to them versus the conformation to societal standards. This activity can be challenging for some, as recalling a time when they felt beautiful may feel inaccessible, so try to use it with a community ready to embrace this powerful discussion. Indicators of readiness include members being able to share positive appraisals of themselves and having moments of positive body image and self-esteem.

When introducing this discussion to the group, explain that feeling beautiful can be elicited by feeling connected to others. When one feels loved, appreciated, and valued by others, it can positively affect their self-image, and as a result they may feel more confident, attractive, and beautiful. When they feel connected to others on a deeper level, such as through shared values, interests, or experiences, they may feel a sense of belonging and acceptance that make them more secure in their own identity and boost their self-esteem, resulting in less concern about conforming to external standards of beauty.

**Begin** the discussion by asking group members to share what comes to mind when they think of conventional beauty standards.

**Ask** members to brainstorm what makes a person beautiful beyond their physical appearance. For example, qualities that can make a person feel beautiful and be beautiful to others may include their personality, character, values, behavior, and actions.

**Prompt** group members:

Share a time you felt beautiful or confident that had nothing to do with your physical appearance.

**Invite** each group member to share their moment.
**Further** the discussion by asking:

- What about this moment or experience allowed you to not focus on your appearance or body?
- How would a preoccupation with your appearance or body have distanced you from how you felt in those moments?
- What would a balance between attending to your appearance and avoiding excessive fixation or self-objectification entail?

**Conclude** by asking group members to identify and share a new conceptualization of beauty informed by this activity and discussion.

### Facilitators' Forum

To take this discussion further, facilitators can ask group members, "Can you identify when you have felt others were beautiful or a moment that was beautiful that had nothing to do with conventional beauty standards, such as 'when I saw my mother's face holding her grandson for the first time'?" This prompt may also be an easier entry point for group members struggling to see themselves as beautiful.

## Activity 8.1 – Diet Culture Mad Libs

Although eating disorder recovery groups can be emotionally intense, injecting humor into the conversations can provide a refreshing shift from the usual group tone. Mad libs are a simple and quick activity that elicits smiles, laughter, and permission to take a step back from serious topics that may feel overwhelming. Humor can help to lighten the mood and infuse lightheartedness into the group.

This activity can also serve as a space-filler if there is some spare time at the end of the group but not enough time to begin a new topic or deep discussion. Facilitators are encouraged to write their own and get creative.

Mad libs could be done as a group, going around in a circle and giving everyone a chance to contribute a word, or facilitators could allow everyone to fill in their own.

## Materials:

- A copy of the mad lib
- For in-person groups, one facilitator will need a writing utensil.
- For virtual groups, one facilitator will need a writing utensil or may use their electronic device.

The following is a sample mad lib about the wellness-obsessed social climate.

This morning I woke up at _____ (time) and made a quick cup of _____ (beverage) and of _____ ("health" food) topped with _____ (spice or herb) and _____ (condiment). It tasted _____ (adjective). I had to rush out the door of my _____ (type of housing) to make it to my _____ (activity) class on time so that I'd feel _____ (adjective) for the rest of the day. But wait! How could I have forgotten to slather my face with my _____ (animal) _____ (body part) extract cream! I'm told it will keep my _____ (body part) from looking _____ (negative adjective). When I went back inside, I got so caught up examining my _____ (body part) in the mirror, this way and that. Then I thought, *maybe*

*I won't go to the class after all.* Instead, I'll stay home and cook up a nice batch of _____ (type of cuisine) _____ ("health" food) for the week. It takes _____ (number) hours, so I'd better get started.

Then I remembered I had _____ (meal of day) plans with my friend, _____ (celebrity). I better wear my _____ (article of clothing) and _____ (type of shoe) from _____ (store) because who knows who we'll see there. I don't even have to look at the menu because I always order _____ (flavor) _____ (a food). It tastes absolutely _____ (adjective). Oh, what a busy day!

## Activity 8.2 – The Recovery Cafe

As a dietitian and a therapist running eating disorder outpatient treatment groups, we understand the importance of providing group members with a safe and supportive environment for recovery. One of our favorite groups we look forward to a few times a year is fondly titled The Recovery Cafe.

The purpose of this activity is twofold. First, we use The Recovery Cafe to introduce group members to books, podcasts, articles, and movies to support their eating disorder recovery. Think book club meets eating disorder group therapy. It gives members some recovery *food for thought* and exposure to resources they might not otherwise know exist. Second, the group provides a safe and supportive environment for members to explore these topics, share their experiences, and challenge their beliefs. By promoting open and constructive discussions on these issues, this activity can help members gain a deeper understanding of themselves and others and facilitate individual growth and healing.

### Choosing Media for the Cafe Group

Group members are often bombarded with an excess of media messages that align with diet culture and may impede their progress in recovery, even if they do not seek out this type of messaging. Diet culture can enter feeds, often disguised as credible health information when in actuality it is sales-oriented product placement coming from someone with no background or education in health or nutrition. This can include following influencers who sometimes post their "what-I-eat-in-a-day" or workout metrics, reading the latest book or blog post about a diet trend, or listening to a podcast that promotes a particular workout app or diet approach. These messages are absorbed and internalized.

Therefore, choosing resources that align with the group's recovery goals is important when selecting media for The Recovery Cafe activity. Facilitators should think about the form and content best suited for their group. In a group of high schoolers already bogged down with homework, suggesting a podcast episode rather than a book may be more realistic. In a group of avid readers, a book may be a welcomed resource.

Select a topic the group could benefit from exploring with different perspectives and research. This information may debunk common beliefs about food and how bodies work. When we select a resource that addresses a stuck point or topic the group seems to return to, the discussion resonates more deeply with everyone.

Finally, time frame and accessibility are important. Facilitators must respect the group members' time and other obligations when requesting that they consume media outside the group. After all, the more group members that read the book, watch the movie, or listen to the podcast in its entirety, the richer the discussion will be.

We often do The Recovery Cafe quarterly. We set a date several weeks in advance (we try to give two months' notice) and ensure the resource is available.

It is helpful to pick media accessible for free or at a low cost. Podcast episodes make great Cafe content because they are free and often short to listen to compared to reading a book. However, a book is an excellent choice and we have frequently utilized them. Remind group members of audiobook options if they do not like or do not have time for reading.

### Group Discussion

Discussion questions will differ depending on the resource used, so group facilitators should prepare before Cafe groups with a list of discussion points. Sometimes discussion guides are available from authors.

While there is no script or questions we can provide since the discussions will go in vastly different directions depending on the resource selected, an effective discussion will cover these questions:

- What were members' reactions to the selected resource?
- Was the information new or a new perspective for them?
- Does consuming this information change their feelings about certain aspects of their recovery?
- Does having consumed this information help them feel less alone in recovery?

## Discussion 8.3: I Spy Diet Culture

One of the challenges of identifying diet culture is that there is no universally accepted definition. However, defining diet culture may help members see how sneaky it is and where it enters their life in ways they did not realize. Facilitators can introduce diet culture by describing it as:

- A societal system that values thinness and equates it with health, beauty, and success
- A belief system that promotes restrictive eating and strict exercise regimens as a means of achieving a certain body size or shape
- A culture that perpetuates the notion that certain foods are "good" or "bad" and that moralizes food choices

- A set of beliefs and behaviors that reinforce weight stigma and discrimination towards individuals in "larger" bodies
- A multibillion-dollar industry that profits off individuals' insecurities and perpetuates the myth of the "perfect" body
- A culture that reinforces harmful gender and race stereotypes related to body size and shape

Through this discussion, members will better understand where diet culture reveals itself and infiltrates day-to-day life. With enhanced awareness of its pervasiveness, members will be equipped to resist these messages more effectively and learn to reject them altogether.

## Materials:

- For in-person groups, consider using a whiteboard with the prompt *Diet culture is . . .* or provide paper and writing utensils for group members.
- For virtual groups, a virtual whiteboard could be used, or ask members to respond in a chat box.

**Begin** by asking members to define diet culture. Let them know there is no official definition. Knowing this may make group members more apt to try defining it.

> Diet culture is . . .

**Ask**:

- How does diet culture show up, such as through advertising, social media, healthcare, and interpersonal interactions?
- What are some catchphrases rooted in diet culture that have entered the vernacular, such as "cleanse" and "cheat day?"
- How would one build resilience against diet culture? How can one exhibit self-compassion when faced with these messages?
- What is the impact of rejecting weight stigma? What could be the benefit of focusing on overall health and well-being (if that is important to you) rather than specific body size or shape?

**Conclude** the group by having group members share something that resonated with them and how it will equip them to protect their recovery as they encounter diet culture "in the wild."

*Facilitators' Forum*

Compile a list of resources that promote body neutrality or positivity, intuitive eating, and a non-diet approach. Offer a variety of resources to cater to different backgrounds, preferences, and needs. These may include books, documentaries, social media accounts, websites, and podcasts. Encourage group members to explore these resources at their own pace and choose the ones that resonate with them. Some of these resources may include:

- Books: Provide a list of recommended books that cover topics such as intuitive eating, body acceptance, and challenging diet culture.
- Documentaries: Suggest documentaries that explore the impact of diet culture, body image, and the importance of self-acceptance. These documentaries can help broaden awareness and promote critical thinking.
- Social media accounts: Recommend influential social media accounts that promote body positivity, intuitive eating, and non-diet approaches. These accounts often share inspirational messages, educational content, and practical tips for navigating healthier relationships with food and the body.
- Websites: Include reputable websites that offer evidence-based information, resources, and support for body acceptance, intuitive eating, and non-diet approaches. These websites may feature articles, blogs, forums, and online communities that provide valuable insights and guidance.
- Podcasts: Suggest podcasts covering topics related to body liberation, intuitive eating, and challenging diet culture. These podcasts often feature interviews, discussions, and expert insights, offering a convenient and accessible way for group members to engage with the material.

## Activity 8.3: Dear Diet Culture

Research findings document the positive experiences of individuals with eating disorders who have participated in therapeutic writing interventions. These findings suggest that emotional expression through writing may help individuals process and cope with difficult emotions while building group cohesion through shared writing activities to foster a sense of support and belonging.[12]

The topic of diet culture can be complex and emotionally charged. Therefore, the intervention of therapeutic letter writing holds special significance. Engaging in the act of writing a letter provides a safe space for participants to express their feelings without the fear of criticism or invalidation. This approach becomes salient for individuals who may feel ashamed or experience stigma regarding their relationship with food and their bodies.

Additionally, writing a therapeutic letter can help group members explore and process their beliefs and values around food and body image. This processing may include identifying ways diet culture has influenced their thinking and behavior and reflecting on alternative perspectives more aligned with their values and eating disorder recovery.

Finally, it can provide a sense of empowerment and agency. By expressing themselves through writing, they can reclaim their narrative, challenge diet culture's harmful and insidious messages, set boundaries, develop greater self-awareness, and cultivate self-acceptance. This activity allows them to assert a new paradigm and identify boundaries to protect themselves or society from the harmful messages and practices it employs.

## Materials:

- Handout "Dear Diet Culture" (Appendix 8A)
- For in-person groups, provide paper and writing utensils for group members.
- For virtual groups, members can gather their writing materials or utilize electronic devices.

**Explain** to the group that they will be doing a therapeutic letter-writing exercise, writing a letter to diet culture as if it were a person. In this letter, group members will express their thoughts, feelings, and experiences related to diet culture. They can share how it has impacted their life, including their relationship with food, body, and sense of self-worth, and feel free to "talk back" to diet culture if they would like. They can even address how it has impacted others they know or society at large.

> Write a letter to diet culture as if it were a person. Express your thoughts, feelings, and experiences related to diet culture.

**Provide** prompts to help guide the letter writing. These prompts can include questions such as:

- How have the cultural and societal messages embedded in diet culture affected your perceptions of health and self-worth?
- How has diet culture contributed to developing or maintaining your eating disorder?
- How has diet culture affected your relationship with food and your body image?
- What messages from diet culture have negatively impacted your life?

- What are some challenges or difficulties that you have faced as a result of diet culture?
- What changes would you like to see in your relationship with diet culture? With society's relationship with diet culture?

If desired, read an example of a letter (Appendix 8A).

**Allow** the group time to write their letters and then encourage them to share the letters.

**Ask** questions to elicit members to share their thoughts and feelings about hearing the letters.

- Did you notice any emotions, thoughts, or physical sensations arise when writing your letter? If so, what did you notice?
- Did you notice any emotions, thoughts, or physical sensations arise when hearing the letters others wrote? If so, what did you notice?
- What is the value of acknowledging and identifying the damaging belief system of diet culture?
- How does one actively unlearn the harmful tenets of diet culture?
- Are there ways individuals can speak out against diet culture when they encounter it?

**Encourage** the group members to reflect on what they can take from the activity and apply it to their recovery.

### Facilitators' Forum

This activity allows one to recognize the worth of emotions, even those considered negative, such as sadness and anger. For example, acknowledging the presence of sadness may enable group members to offer themselves compassion, especially when reflecting on how damaging messages from the diet industry may have affected their well-being, time, and focus. Another example is anger, which has the potential to serve as a strong motivator, compelling group members to take action toward creating change. For instance, an individual may choose to unfollow a social media influencer who endorses diet culture in response to their anger.

## Activity 8.4: Taking a Stand

Unlike the therapeutic letter to diet culture, which is a personal exploration primarily focused on the group members' growth and reflection, writing a letter targeting entities that profit off diet culture is an act of advocacy focused on promoting societal change. This type of letter writing can also develop a feeling of empowerment, connection, and purpose while also building assertiveness skills.

## Materials:

- Handout "Taking a Stand" (Appendix 8B)
- For in-person groups, provide paper and writing utensils for group members.
- For virtual groups, members can gather their writing materials or utilize electronic devices.

**Explain** to the group that they will be doing a letter-writing exercise where they write letters to businesses, industries, or professionals who spread harmful messages that promote unrealistic and homogeneous body ideals, restrictive or fad diets, or weight stigma. Group members can decide whether or not they want to send the letters; this activity has therapeutic value regardless of their decision.

> Write a letter to a business, industry, or professional who has spread harmful messages that promote unrealistic and homogenous body ideals, restrictive or fad diets, or weight stigma.

**Offer** the group a set of prompts to help guide their letter writing. These prompts can include questions such as:

- Can you identify some companies, industries, or professionals promoting harmful and discriminatory messages about physical appearance or unattainable physical standards? How about some that engage in weight bias?
- Can you identify some companies, industries, or professionals that promote restrictive or fad diets?
- Do these companies, industries, or professionals profit from your eating disorder? If so, how?
- Have these businesses, industries, or professionals contributed to your body image dissatisfaction? Have they contributed to feelings of body shame and led to the development of your eating disorder? Have they impacted your eating disorder recovery?
- What messages would you like to send to these businesses, industries, or professionals about the harmful effects of the messages they are promoting?
- What changes would you like to see in the advertising and marketing strategies of these businesses, industries, or professionals? Examples include having a diverse representation of bodies, more inclusive sizing of clothes, and refraining from promoting diets.
- How can businesses, industries, and professionals become more inclusive and representative of body diversity?

**Provide** group members with letter templates, which can be found in Appendix 8B, which they can use, modify, or create an original. Give ample time to compose their letters.

**Give** group members the option to share their letters with the group. Facilitators may use the following questions regarding the process and content of this activity to further the discussion.

- Was it easy to identify a business, industry, or professional to write to? If not, why?
- Did your message at the end of your letter writing match what you expected to write, or did your letter evolve in a different way than you expected?
- What was it like to hear other group members' letters? Did you notice feeling any strong emotions as you listened to them?

### Facilitators' Forum

To expand on this discussion, facilitators may encourage group members to brainstorm other ideas about how the group can take action to advocate against businesses, industries, or professionals that promote discriminatory and dangerous messages about food and bodies. Some ideas may include:

- Sending their letters or starting a letter-writing campaign
- Writing reviews or comments on social media or review platforms
- Supporting businesses and industries that promote diverse and realistic body representation
- Unfollowing social media accounts whose posts promote diet culture
- Joining a body positivity or acceptance campaign or charity that encourages going beyond superficial body standards

## Media Literacy

We are constantly bombarded with messages from the media, both overtly and covertly, that dictate how we should look and feel. These messages try to sell us products and services with promises of health, happiness, eternal youth, and true love. As a result, many feel compelled to diet, exercise excessively, take supplements, purchase expensive serums and creams, or even undergo surgery. Moreover, if the consumer fails to achieve the advertised results, it can lead to feelings of shame, self-blame, and impaired self-esteem. It is often seen as a personal failure rather than a systemic problem created and perpetuated by diet culture.

The rise of social media has transformed the advertising landscape. Advertisements are now more insidious, and it can be difficult to differentiate them from standard content. Influencers may endorse particular products, sometimes disclosing that it is an #ad or #sponsored, but not always.

While media does not cause eating disorders, media contributes to body dissatisfaction, promoting weight loss practices and encouraging the internalization of the "thin ideal." These are established risk factors for the development of eating disorders.[13]

The goal of media literacy goes beyond recognizing digital editing and other forms of image manipulation.[14] It aims to empower individuals to evaluate media content critically, enabling them to identify, analyze, and challenge it. Over time, practicing media literacy builds one's ability to propose alternative perspectives to harmful, stereotypical messages commonly conveyed through mass media.[15] This approach empowers individuals to make informed choices regarding media consumption and creation.

### Activity 8.5 – Mastering the Media

In the first part of this activity, the group will closely examine the concept of media literacy. This will include defining the term, identifying the skills necessary to practice it, and providing group members a chance to evaluate media messages using this framework.

The second part of this activity involves asking group members to identify how media messages perpetuate diet culture. The facilitators ask participants to recognize how these messages can mimic the negative internal voice that individuals with eating disorders experience and their role in contributing to social injustice. Additionally, members are prompted to explore how advertisers can get away with disseminating these messages and why they are successful.

### Materials:

- Handout "Media Literacy Guide" (Appendix 8C)
- Media content provided by group facilitators

**Share** the "Media Literacy Guide" (Appendix 8C) and the media content provided by group facilitators. The media content should illustrate objectification and sexualization of bodies (i.e., showing body parts), the lack of diversity in representation, giving mixed messages (i.e., promoting a diet while also promoting spontaneity), equating weight loss with finding a partner, having a "happy" life, etc. (Advertisements on television, the internet, social media, and magazine content can serve as excellent resources for analyzing how media can create and perpetuate insecurities to sell products and services.)

**Evaluate** the media content using the questions on the "Media Literacy Guide."

**Encourage** discussion about ways group members can actively resist and push back against unhealthy messages in their own lives. This resistance could include strategies like unfollowing social media accounts that promote unrealistic beauty standards, avoiding conversations or activities that promote disordered eating, or seeking out alternative perspectives and voices within the media.

*Part Two: Discussion*

**Begin** by asking group members if they feel media messages contribute to the perpetuation of diet culture, including contributing to and maintaining their eating disorder, and if so, how.

**Ask** the group:

> How do media messages mimic the negative internal voice that individuals with eating disorders experience? What roles do these messages play in contributing to social injustice?

**Prompt** members to explore how advertisers can get away with disseminating these messages and why they are successful by asking:

- How can you identify diet culture messages in advertising, social media, and other forms of media?
- What signs or phrases might indicate that a message promotes harmful diet culture beliefs?
- What is the value of having media literacy?

*Facilitators' Forum*

Facilitators can enrich this discussion by exploring the concept of intersectionality, which refers to the interconnected nature of various aspects of an individual's identity and its relationship with media influence. In this context, intersectionality acknowledges that a person's experiences are shaped by multiple factors, such as race, gender, sexuality, physical abilities, and socioeconomic status, which intersect and interact with each other.

By guiding group members to understand this concept, facilitators can help participants recognize how media influences do not operate in isolation but intersect with different facets of their lives. For example, a member's racial or ethnic background may intersect with media portrayals of beauty standards, leading to complex feelings about body image and self-acceptance.

Encouraging participants to delve into how these interconnected identities shape their experiences with media and body image will lead to a more meaningful and comprehensive conversation. Participants may share personal stories, like how gender representation in media impacts their perception of body image or how media messages about socioeconomic status influence their self-worth. This understanding will enable them to develop more nuanced and empowering strategies for navigating media messages, fostering positive self-image and resilience in the face of societal pressures.

## Notes

1   Harrison, Christy. 2018. *"What Is Diet Culture?" Christy Harrison - Intuitive Eating Dietitian, Anti-Diet Author, & Certified Eating Disorders Specialist*, August 10, 2018. https://christyharrison.com/blog/what-is-diet-culture.
2   Harrison, "What Is Diet Culture," 2018.
3   Stice, Eric, Carolyn Black Becker, and Sonja Yokum. 2013. "Eating Disorder Prevention: Current Evidence-Base and Future Directions." *International Journal of Eating Disorders* 46 (5): 478–485. https://doi.org/10.1002/eat.22105.
4   Piran, Niva. 2017. *Journeys of Embodiment at the Intersection of Body and Culture the Developmental Theory of Embodiment.* Saint Louis: Elsevier Science.
5   Tylka, Tracy L. 2019. "Broad Conceptualization of Beauty." Essay. In *Handbook of Positive Body Image and Embodiment: Constructs, Protective Factors, and Interventions*, edited by Tracy L. Tylka and Niva Piran. New York: Oxford University Press. https://doi.org/10.1093/med-psych/9780190841874.001.0001.
6   Buote, Vanessa M., Anne E. Wilson, Erin J. Strahan, Stephanie B. Gazzola, and Fiona Papps. 2011. "Setting the Bar: Divergent Sociocultural Norms for Women's and Men's Ideal Appearance in Real-World Contexts." *Body Image* 8 (4): 322–334. https://doi.org/10.1016/j.bodyim.2011.06.002.
7   Piran, *Journeys of Embodiment*, 2017.
8   Kinsey, Dalia. 2022. *Decolonizing Wellness a QTBIPOC-Centered Guide to Escape the Diet Trap, Heal Your Self-Image, and Achieve Body Liberation*, 107. New York: BenBella Books.
9   Stice, Eric, and Heather E. Shaw. 2002. "Role of Body Dissatisfaction in the Onset and Maintenance of Eating Pathology." *Journal of Psychosomatic Research* 53 (5): 985–993. https://doi.org/10.1016/s0022-3999(02)00488-9.
10  Tylka, "Broad Conceptualization of Beauty," 2019.
11  Tylka, 2019.
12  Ramsey-Wade, Christine E., Heidi Williamson, and Jane Meyrick. 2020. "Therapeutic Writing for Disordered Eating: A Systematic Review." *Journal of Creativity in Mental Health* 16 (1): 59–76. https://doi.org/10.1080/15401383.2020.1760988.
13  Holland, Grace, and Marika Tiggemann. 2016. "A Systematic Review of the Impact of the Use of Social Networking Sites on Body Image and Disordered Eating Outcomes." *Body Image* 17: 100–110. https://doi.org/10.1016/j.bodyim.2016.02.008.
14  Cash, T. F., and Pruzinsky, T. 2002. "Future Challenges for Body Image Theory, Research, and Clinical Practice." In *Body Images: A Handbook of Theory, Research, and Clinical Practice*, edited by T. F. Cash and T. Pruzinsky, 509–516. New York: Guilford Press.
15  Levine, Michael P., Niva Piran, and Charlie Stoddard. 1999. "Mission More Probable: Media Literacy, Activism and Advocacy as Primary Prevention." Essay. In *Preventing Eating Disorders: A Handbook of Interventions and Special Challenges*, edited by Niva Piran, Michael P. Levine, and Catherine Steiner-Adair, 3–25. London: Routledge.

# Appendix 8A – Dear Diet Culture (for Activity 8.3)

Dear Diet Culture,

I am writing to express my frustration, anger, and disappointment in how you have impacted my life. I have been caught up in your never-ending cycle of restriction, guilt, and shame for years.

You convinced me that the only way to be happy and healthy was to be thin, and I spent years chasing after this unattainable ideal. I deprived myself of food, I exercised obsessively, and I punished myself when I inevitably fell off the wagon. But now, I am seeing the damage that you have done. I see the toll your messages have taken on my mental and physical health. I am tired of feeling guilty whenever I eat something you deem "bad." I am tired of punishing myself with grueling workouts that leave me exhausted and depleted.

I am learning to reject your messages and embrace a more compassionate, intuitive approach to eating and movement. I am learning to listen to my body's cues and to honor my hunger and fullness. I am learning to move my body in ways that feel good, rather than punishing myself for not adhering to your rigid standards.

I am done with your harmful messages. I am done with the way you have impacted my life. I am reclaiming my power and my health, and I am refusing to let you dictate my worth.

Sincerely,

An individual who is done with your harmful influence

Dear Diet Culture,

While I have considered our relationship over a long time ago, that hasn't stopped you from showing up everywhere and sweet-talking others with your promise of a "happily ever after" that can never exist with you. I see you as trying to hide behind new identities, calling yourself "wellness," "health," or "clean eating" in an attempt to attract new followers. Make no mistake, you are the same manipulative force you have always been. I've seen you take advantage of people by preying on their insecurities and fears, making false promises, and leaving them feeling like they are the problem. You profit off their pain and suffering, all while convincing them that it is for their own good. You are the ultimate gaslighter.

I refuse to be a part of your game anymore. I know that my worth is not determined by the size or shape of my body, and I will no longer let you convince me otherwise. I will not let you make me feel guilty for enjoying food or for taking a break from exercising. I am learning to listen to my body and take care of myself in a nurturing and sustainable way.

While I may not be able to stop you single-handedly, be warned I am not alone. Many others like me see through your lies and refuse to be manipulated by you. We are fighting back against your harmful influence. You were socially constructed, far from being a universal truth.

So, Diet Culture, consider this a warning. We are onto you and see you through all your disguises. You may have had a grip on us for a while, but we are stronger than you think.

Sincerely,

An individual who is done playing your games

# Appendix 8B – Taking a Stand (for Activity 8.4)

Dear [Retailer],

I am writing to express my concern regarding exclusively using images featuring only extremely thin, white, and able-bodied women in your advertising. These images promote an unhealthy and unrealistic body ideal that can contribute to eating disorders and other negative health outcomes.

As a consumer, I value your company's products and services. However, I am troubled by the message that these images send to women and girls, particularly those who may already be struggling with body image issues or eating disorders. Research has shown that exposure to unrealistic beauty standards can increase body dissatisfaction and disordered eating behaviors.

I understand that as a retailer, you are responsible for selling products and promoting your brand. However, more responsible ways exist without contributing to harmful attitudes toward food, weight, and body image. I urge you to consider using more diverse and inclusive imagery in your advertising, that better reflects the diversity of your customers and promotes healthy and positive attitudes towards body image.

Thank you for taking the time to consider my concerns. I look forward to seeing positive changes in your advertising in the future.

Sincerely,

[Your name]

Dear [Doctor],

I am writing to express my concern about the promotion of restrictive diets or weight loss as a medical intervention. These practices can be harmful and contribute to the development of eating disorders and other negative health outcomes.

I understand that as a healthcare provider, you have a responsibility to promote the health and well-being of your patients. However, I am troubled by the message that these practices send to individuals who may already be struggling with body image issues or disordered eating behaviors. Research has shown that dieting and weight loss interventions can negatively affect physical and mental health, including increased risk of eating disorders, weight cycling, and decreased self-esteem.

I urge you to consider alternative approaches that focus on promoting healthy habits and positive attitudes towards food and body image rather than promoting restrictive diets or weight loss as a primary goal. This may include promoting intuitive eating, physical activity for enjoyment, and other healthful behaviors that do not rely on the pursuit of specific body weight or size.

Thank you for taking the time to consider my concerns. I believe that as a healthcare provider, you have the power to make a positive impact on the lives of your patients and promote health and well-being in a responsible and sustainable way.

Sincerely,

[Your name]

# Appendix 8C – Media Literacy Guide (for Activity 8.5)

## Assess

- How might the message make someone feel about themselves?
- How might the message make someone feel about other people – friends, family members, someone they see at the store or online, etc...?
- How does the message perpetuate or challenge diet culture and social injustice?

## Reflect

- What does the message mean to you?
- Does it reinforce or conflict with your work in eating disorder recovery?
- Does it make you want to change something about yourself?

## Evaluate

- Who created and profits from this message?
- What is the message trying to convey, and what values or beliefs does it promote?
- What is their agenda? Is it to inform, entertain, persuade, or some combination of these? Is it to gain power, profit, or influence?
- What assumptions or biases are underlying the message?
- Who is the target audience?
- What is left out of the message?
- What is the tone of the message? Is it using fear or shame to elicit interest in the product/service?
- Are there any images or visuals accompanying the message? Do these images accurately represent a diverse range of body types and sizes, or do they promote a narrow and unrealistic beauty standard? Are there any signs of alteration/digital manipulation that may create unrealistic expectations or perpetuate harmful appearance ideals?
- If applicable, what claims are being made in the message? Are these claims backed up by scientific evidence or research, or are they based on personal anecdotes or opinions?

*Figure 8.1* A diagram indicating questions to ask oneself to evaluate, determine the impact of, and reflect on diet culture's impact on media.

# Chapter 9

## Nurturing Body Image and Embracing Embodiment

### Elevating Body Image Work with Group Therapy

Body image disturbances are widely recognized as enduring features commonly observed in individuals diagnosed with eating disorders. The diagnostic criteria for Anorexia Nervosa and Bulimia Nervosa include the influence of body shape or weight on self-evaluation.[1] While body image is traditionally conceptualized as a mental representation, contemporary research suggests that it encompasses various dimensions beyond a simple mental picture of the body.[2]

Eating disorders often involve a complex interplay between emotions and the body. Negative perceptions or views of one's body can arise when individuals ignore or disregard their internal signals and emotions. Instead of paying attention to their internal experiences, one may rely heavily on external appearance to regulate emotions or cope with these internal struggles. Moving beyond a one-dimensional perspective is crucial to address the complexity of body image and embodiment.[3]

This chapter provides facilitators with tools to address body image and embodiment in the context of eating disorder recovery. Acknowledging that body image encompasses sensory and emotional aspects, and that participants may struggle to verbalize them effectively, experiential approaches are introduced as an alternative way to establish a profound connection with the body. These approaches are informed by the knowledge that body image development begins in a preverbal stage.[4] Therefore, methods that bypass the limitations of verbal expression are provided.

The somatic techniques that will be introduced include body awareness exercises and mental representation approaches, such as journal writing and guided imagery. By engaging in these activities, individuals in eating disorder recovery can directly experience alternative ways to address their challenges and discover potential paths to healing.

In addition to experiential approaches, this chapter incorporates principles from Cognitive Behavioral Therapy (CBT), Dialectical Behavior Therapy (DBT), and Acceptance Commitment Therapy (ACT). By drawing on these therapeutic modalities, facilitators can provide a comprehensive framework for supporting group members to embrace embodiment and foster healthier

DOI: 10.4324/9781003430964-12

relationships with their bodies. These evidence-based techniques and strategies help group members challenge negative thought patterns, develop effective coping skills, cultivate self-compassion, and practice accepting their bodies as they progress in their recovery.

## Mindfulness for Improving Body Image and Embodiment

Mindfulness-based interventions are effective in nurturing greater attentiveness toward internal experiences in the present moment and reducing critical judgments regarding appearance, both directed toward oneself and others.[5] Studies show these interventions reduce reactivity to body-related thoughts and emotions while promoting a compassionate relationship with oneself and the body.[6]

Often, one responds to body image distress by avoiding those uncomfortable thoughts or feelings or ruminating on them. Avoidance may include wearing baggy clothing to prevent the sensation of fabric touching the body or avoiding a mirror to circumvent seeing one's reflection. These sensations, thoughts, and ensuing feelings trigger body image distress. Conversely, someone may become hyperfocused on a body image thought, feeling, or sensation. Both responses will prevent them from having the ability to be present. It follows that cultivating mindfulness skills is critical in body image work and thus in recovery.

The following three exercises utilize mindfulness to help group members connect with their bodies, cultivate awareness, and build self-trust.

## Discussion 9.1: A Case for Mindfulness

This discussion aims to educate group members about the advantages of practicing mindfulness instead of avoiding or ruminating when dealing with body image distress. Sharing experiences with these practices will help group members normalize the challenges inherent in mindfulness and increase the willingness to try them.

**Begin** by providing education about the connection between mindfulness and body image.

**Ask** group members to share how they currently cope with body image distress. What are the downsides or limitations of those strategies?

**Help** members label behaviors as avoidance or rumination to help draw a clear distinction between those and a mindfulness approach. Group members are encouraged to share their experiences and challenges with avoidance behaviors.

**Highlight** the connection between mindfulness, body awareness, and fostering a more compassionate relationship with oneself. To guide the discussion toward recognizing the need for alternative approaches that promote present-moment awareness and self-compassion, facilitators can ask:

Can you share a time when mindfulness (being in the present moment) helped you tolerate body image distress?

**Further** the discussion by asking:

- What gets in the way of using mindfulness before resorting to rumination or avoidance?
- Are there any potential risks or side effects associated with using mindfulness in certain contexts?
- What are some practical strategies to integrate mindfulness into daily life and make it a habit?

### Facilitators' Forum

Group members may bring up using distraction as a strategy to cope with body image distress. While distraction can effectively allow the distress to naturally subside over time, it is crucial to emphasize the importance of mindfulness in this process. Mindfulness involves remaining aware of negative body image thoughts and the urge to engage in behaviors in response to those thoughts while consciously redirecting attention to other activities or thoughts. By incorporating mindfulness, individuals can cultivate greater self-awareness and make intentional choices in managing their body image concerns.

## Activity 9.1 – 3 Minute Breathing Space for Body Image

The 3 Minute Breathing Space technique is a brief mindfulness practice developed by Zindel Segal, John Teasdale, and Mark Williams, the creators of Mindfulness-Based Cognitive Therapy (MBCT).[7] This exercise aims to support participants to consciously enter the present moment and observe one's thoughts and sensations without judgment. Doing so supports a gradual shift in mindset, fostering a more supportive and nurturing attitude toward one's body. Regular engagement in this practice can cultivate greater self-acceptance and compassion, leading to a healthier and more positive relationship with oneself. This exercise holds particular value when individuals experience negative thoughts about their bodies, as these thoughts often initiate a chain reaction of self-criticism and distress. The process involves three steps: cultivating awareness, focusing attention, and expanding awareness.

Facilitators may use the following script to guide group members through this mini-meditation. Feel free to adapt and customize these instructions according to your preferences and group needs.

**Introduce** this adapted version of the 3 Minute Breathing Space specifically tailored for the group to focus on embodiment and body image. This mindfulness practice aims to help group members cultivate a deeper connection with their bodies and develop a more positive and compassionate relationship with their physical selves. By engaging in this practice, group members can increase their awareness of sensations, thoughts, and emotions related to their bodies without judgment or criticism.

**Ask** group members to find a comfortable position. If the group is in person, this may be a seated position or lying on their backs if the space allows for that. For virtual groups, encourage group members to find a comfortable position in their space. Invite group members to close their eyes if they would like.

**Use** the following script:

**Step One: Grounding in the Body** Begin by bringing your attention to the physical sensations in your body. Notice the contact of your body with the chair or floor. Feel the support beneath you. Tune in to the subtle sensations, such as warmth, tingling, or any areas of tension or relaxation. Allow yourself to fully inhabit your body in this present moment.

**Step Two: Exploring Body Awareness** Shift your attention to the sensations in your body, particularly focusing on the areas related to body image concerns. Notice any tightness, discomfort, or areas of tension. Observe without judgment or the need to change anything. Simply acknowledge the sensations and emotions that arise without getting caught up in them.

**Step Three: Expanding Awareness with Compassion** Expand your awareness to include your thoughts and emotions related to your body image. Notice any self-critical or negative thoughts that arise or any sensations of discomfort, tension, or resistance. Instead of getting carried away by these thoughts or sensations, observe them without judgment and consciously breathe into those areas as you inhale. Then, as you exhale, release and soften any tension, allowing for a sense of openness and self-compassion. Practice observing them with compassion and gentleness. Cultivate self-acceptance and kindness toward your body, embracing its uniqueness and inherent value.

**Invite** group members to open their eyes and give themselves a warm hug and thank themselves for their willingness to participate in this activity. Allow group members to share their experiences with this meditation and encourage regular practice to elicit a more peaceful and present relationship with their bodies and themselves.

**Further** the discussion with these questions:

• What challenges did you experience as you engaged in this meditation? How did you try to work through them?

- Can you imagine yourself using this meditation in your day-to-day life? Why or why not?
- What sensations did you notice in your body as you engaged in this meditation? What thoughts did you observe?
- Did you notice areas of your body where you have body image distress, and could you detach from that? How did that feel?

### Facilitators' Forum

Including a mindful transition at the beginning of this or any other mindfulness activity can be beneficial. This transition entails guiding group members in shifting from their everyday mindset to the meditation practice. Incorporate mindful transitions, such as a brief body scan or gentle stretching, to help them fully arrive in the present moment and cultivate awareness of their bodies before starting the 3 Minute Breathing Space.

## Compassion-Based Interventions

Compassion-based interventions target the detrimental effects of shame and self-criticism associated with pathological body image dissatisfaction. These interventions aim to foster a sense of acceptance and kindness toward oneself when faced with distressing body image concerns. Empirical research has shown that incorporating self-compassion meditations into treatment can yield positive outcomes by reducing maladaptive body processes, including self-criticism, body dissatisfaction, eating pathology, and appearance comparison; additionally, these interventions promote beneficial processes such as body appreciation and flexibility in one's perception of body image.[8]

## Activity 9.2 – Compassionate Body Scan

The compassionate body scan is a technique that can improve body image by fostering a greater sense of connection, awareness, and acceptance of one's body. It involves mentally "scanning" or exploring the body from head to toe, paying attention to any sensations, feelings, and physical experiences in each area with compassionate awareness. By using imagination, one can bring awareness to the external aspects of the body, such as warmth, tension, or tingling sensations. It allows participants to deepen their connection with their physical selves and better understand how their bodies express themselves in the present moment.

This activity also promotes a nonreactive and accepting stance, fostering a compassionate and nonjudgmental attitude toward one's body. Facilitators incorporate self-compassion into the body scan by encouraging group members to treat themselves with kindness and care.

The body scan encourages acknowledging and accepting the body as it is, cultivating gratitude for its resilience, functionality, and capacity to experience sensations, leading to a more positive and appreciative attitude toward one's body.

A sample script is provided to get group facilitators started with setting the tone for the activity and beginning with the first region of the body. Group facilitators should continue up the body, using whichever body regions they would like to use from the provided list.

**Introduce** the activity, and provide education regarding the rationale behind this intervention, specifically how it can improve body image.

* For an in-person group, if the environment allows, invite group members to lie down if they prefer that to a sitting position. Members can choose to lie down for virtual groups if they can still hear the facilitator's prompts.
* If group members are experiencing any judgments or negative associations with a specific body part or they are experiencing physical discomfort, they can consider placing a hand on that area as an act of kindness, release tension, and allow that area to soften as if that body part were wrapped in a warm towel. Address any sensations with kind words, such as "There's a little discomfort there, and it's okay for now." They can alternatively transition to another part if the discomfort feels too great.

**Use** (or modify) the script:

Begin the Compassionate Body Scan by finding a comfortable position. You can lie on your back with your palms facing up and feet slightly apart or sit on a comfortable chair with your feet resting on the floor.

Embrace a sense of stillness as you find your place in the present moment, and if necessary, make any subtle adjustments with gentle awareness to ensure your comfort throughout the exercise. If it feels right for you, softly close your eyes and take a few deep breaths, fully immersing yourself in the present moment.

Now, let's bring attention to the breath. Notice the gentle rhythm of your breathing, the sensation of inhaling and exhaling. There's no need to change your breath. Simply hold a compassionate awareness of your breath as it flows naturally.

Shift your focus to your body. Begin to notice how it feels, the gentle touch of your clothing against your skin, the supportive surface beneath you, and the temperature of your body and the environment around you.

As we continue, let's cultivate self-compassion by turning attention to any bodily sensations. Notice areas that may be tingling, sore, or feeling heavy or light. Also, pay attention to any areas that lack sensation or feel hypersensitive. Approach these sensations with gentleness and non-judgment.

Now, let's begin by directing your attention to your feet. Notice any sensations in this area, such as warmth, tingling, or tension. Simply feel the feelings in your feet – ease, discomfort, or perhaps nothing at all – and allow each sensation to be as it is. Take a moment to appreciate your feet's hard work supporting your entire body throughout the day. Offer an inner smile of recognition or appreciation to your feet.

Moving up to your ankles and lower legs, continue to observe any sensations and offer words of compassion to yourself. Allow any tension or discomfort to soften with each breath.

**Guide** group members to move through the body in the following, or desired, order. Include recognition of what each body part does for the person and what they might appreciate about the functionality of that body part.

1. Feet
2. Ankles
3. Lower legs
4. Knees
5. Thighs
6. Hips and pelvic region (buttocks, tailbone, etc.)
7. Abdomen
8. Lower back
9. Chest and ribs
10. Upper back and shoulder blades
11. Hands (fingers, palms, backs, wrists)
12. Arms (lower, elbows, upper arms)
13. Neck
14. Face and head (jaw, mouth, nose, cheeks, ears, eyes, forehead, scalp, back and top of the head)

**Ask** group members to gently shift their attention back to their breath, slowly open their eyes, and return to the room, nurturing a sense of self-care and compassion.

**Reflect** on their experience during the body scan, asking them to share any insights, challenges, or emotions that arose during this activity by asking:

• When this activity was introduced, did you have any preconceived notions or expectations about it? If so, what were they?
• As you went through the activity, did you notice anything about your body that surprised you? If so, could you explain what it was and how it impacted your experience?
• After completing the activity, do you feel a softened attitude toward your body, possibly self-acceptance or gratitude? If so, could you elaborate on the changes you have noticed in your perception and acceptance of your body?
• In what situations or circumstances would you find it beneficial to use a compassionate body scan in your life?

*Facilitators' Forum*

Progressive Muscle Relaxation is another valuable tool for improving one's relationship with their body and can be an alternate or additional activity to practice in the group setting. Like the compassionate body scan, it can increase body awareness, release tension, reduce anxiety, and promote calm and well-being.

## Body Functionality and Appreciation

Body functionality refers to the diverse capabilities and functions of the human body, including physical capacities, health, internal processes, senses, creative endeavors, self-care, and communication with others.[9,10] It emphasizes what the body can do rather than its appearance or perceived flaws, promoting a comprehensive perspective that includes individuals of all abilities.[11]

Research consistently demonstrates that prioritizing body functionality is associated with increased body satisfaction among adult women, as well as adolescent girls and boys; this emphasis on functionality fosters acceptance of perceived imperfections, reduces the internalization of appearance-related messages, and diminishes the importance placed on media ideals and comments about one's appearance.[12,13] The focus on body functionality acts as a protective factor against the impact of diet culture messaging and negative body talk.

Moreover, prioritizing body functionality is linked to greater body appreciation, characterized by unconditional approval and respect for the body.[14] Body appreciation has a stronger positive impact on body image and overall well-being compared to mere satisfaction with physical appearance.[15]

Conversely, self-objectification, which involves viewing oneself primarily as an object to be looked at, is associated with body surveillance, disordered eating attitudes and behaviors, and negative body image.[16,17] Emphasizing body functionality is correlated with lower levels of self-objectification.[18,19] Engaging in physical activities that prioritize body functionality rather than focusing on weight loss or aesthetics also helps reduce self-objectification.[20,21,22]

In summary, embracing body functionality promotes greater body appreciation, protects against self-objectification, and positively influences body image and overall well-being.

## Activity 9.3 – Embracing Body Functionality

## Materials:

- Worksheet "Exploring Body Functionality" (Appendix 9A)
- For in-person groups, provide paper and writing utensils for group members.
- For virtual groups, members can gather their writing materials or utilize electronic devices for the activity.

**Begin** by explaining the concept of body functionality and its importance in fostering a positive body image and overall well-being. Emphasize that body functionality encompasses a wide range of capabilities and abilities beyond physical appearance.

**Allow** time for group members to fill out the worksheet for this activity (Appendix 9A).

**Provide** opportunities for group members to share their thoughts, ask questions, and engage in a discussion about their responses on the worksheet.

**Encourage** group members to take a moment and reflect on these responses and overall experience completing this worksheet. Ask them to consider how focusing on the functions of their body and its capabilities may impact their perspective of body image and self-acceptance. The following questions can help further the discussion.

- How has this activity helped you shift your focus from appearance to body functionality?
- What new insights or appreciation do you have for your body after exploring its functions?
- How can you integrate this knowledge into your daily life to improve body image and overall well-being?

### Facilitators' Forum

Facilitators can prompt group members to consider whether they find their loved ones less lovable or reject them as they grow and change. This inquiry is a powerful parallel to challenge participants' perceptions of their bodies. By posing this question, facilitators encourage participants to question why their relationship with their bodies should differ. It prompts them to reflect on the impact of unrealistic and unnatural standards. It encourages them to embrace self-acceptance and unconditional love for their bodies throughout their own growth and change. By stimulating this introspection, facilitators can support participants to reevaluate their relationships with their bodies and nurture a healthier and more compassionate connection with themselves.

## Discussion 9.2 – Embrace Your Body: A Visualization

Through self-reflection and examination of thought patterns, group members can gain insights into the influence of weight, shape, and appearance on their self-evaluation. The goal is to identify and reframe negative thoughts, paving the way for more positive and empowering perspectives.

Encouraging participants to observe their thoughts and emotions without judgment creates an opportunity to develop a more present-moment awareness of their bodily experiences. This approach supports group members in accepting their feelings and building skills to cope with distress without using the eating disorder.

Through ACT techniques, individuals can develop greater psychological flexibility, allowing them to make choices aligned with their values and move toward a more positive relationship with their body.

**Begin** by asking the prompt:

> When envisioning your ideal relationship with your body, how would you describe it?
> What qualities and characteristics would you like to cultivate?

**Ask** group members to reflect on their current relationship with their body and ask, *How far are you from achieving this desired relationship with your body?*
**Further** the discussion by asking:

- Can you improve your relationship with your body at your current weight or shape? Is it contingent upon meeting specific criteria, such as reaching a certain weight or measurement?
- For those who have already achieved a neutral or positive body image, do you feel that it is dependent on your body remaining unchanged? If so, consider the origins of those conditions. Where do they come from, and how do they impact your ability to foster a peaceful relationship with your body?

**Brainstorm** some strategies for improving members' relationships with their bodies that do not involve engaging in eating disorder behaviors. What alternative approaches are they willing to explore to nurture a healthier connection with their bodies?

- An example may be a member wanting to be more attuned to their body's signals and needs. Attunement for them involves listening to their body's cues for hunger, fullness, fatigue, and pain and responding to them with care and understanding.
- Another example may be wanting to approach their body with more gratitude and mindfulness. This stance may involve recognizing all the amazing things their body allows them to do and experience. They may see practicing mindfulness as a way to help them stay present in their body, appreciating each moment, and fostering a deeper connection with themselves.

### Facilitators' Forum

To enrich this discussion, the dietitian can provide education about set-point weight theory, which posits that the human body strives to maintain a weight within a predetermined range. Understanding and accepting one's set-point range is considered a crucial aspect of eating disorder recovery, as constantly attempting to manipulate weight downward perpetuates the continuation of eating disorder behaviors. Encouraging group members to envision a positive or peaceful connection with their bodies can prompt them to contemplate their own set-point range, representing a weight range that participants can maintain without resorting to harmful eating disorder behaviors. This shift in perspective fosters a focus on overall well-being and supports individuals in cultivating a healthy relationship with their bodies and nourishment.

## Expanding Perspectives: Exploring Diverse Approaches to Body Image Work

There are various approaches to exploring body image, including body positivity, body neutrality, and radical acceptance. Each of these approaches offers valuable perspectives and has its own merits. It is important to provide diverse paradigms because individuals may resonate with different frameworks based on their unique experiences and needs. Additionally, while a specific approach may have been beneficial for someone in the past, they may discover that a different approach is more relevant and meaningful at their current stage of recovery. Flexibility and openness to exploring different perspectives can enhance the effectiveness of body image work.

### Body Positivity

Body positivity is a social movement and ideology that promotes acceptance and appreciation of all bodies, regardless of size, shape, or appearance. It encourages individuals to embrace their bodies and the diversity of bodies around them, rejecting societal beauty standards and norms that perpetuate body shaming and discrimination. Body positivity aims to foster self-love, self-acceptance, and a positive body image while challenging body stereotypes and promoting inclusivity, equality, and respect for all bodies. It emphasizes that all bodies are worthy of love, respect, and dignity, regardless of societal judgments or expectations.

In her book *Fat Talk: Parenting in the Age of Diet Culture*, journalist Virginia Sole-Smith summarizes how body positivity is rooted in second-wave feminism but has experienced a major revival in the past decade, largely through social media and retail marketing endeavors.[23] Body image work through a body-positive lens may look like asking someone what they appreciate about a body part they are self-conscious about or using activities that emphasize what someone likes or appreciates about their body.

While body positivity is transformational for some, many people who struggle with eating disorders unsurprisingly find it difficult. Body positivity assumes that a person can appreciate their body or see it as satisfactory, perhaps even beautiful, just as it is. This approach may not feel within reach for someone grappling to accept their body weight, shape, or size.

### Body Neutrality

Body neutrality emerged as a response to body positivity. This approach emphasizes shifting the focus away from appearance and external judgments of the body, asserting that one need not love or embrace their body; rather, the body is a neutral entity that deserves to be accepted. It encourages individuals to appreciate their bodies for their functionality, resilience, and the experiences they enable rather than solely focusing on aesthetics. Body neutrality promotes self-care practices that prioritize physical and mental well-being rather than pursuing unrealistic beauty standards or seeking external validation based on appearance.

Body neutrality resonates with so many people with eating disorders because it does not require that someone love their body – something that many people who struggle with eating disorders do not feel capable of at certain points in their recovery. Instead, focusing on how someone feels in their body and what their body is capable of may be much more salient than the expectation that they suddenly love and appreciate their body. This functional approach is a natural precursor for encouraging individualized self-care and understanding of our body's inherent worth.

### Radical Acceptance

Psychologist and DBT developer Marsha Linehan coined the term "radical acceptance" in 1993.[24] Rooted in Buddhist beliefs, this approach has been applied to many topics, including body image. In the context of body image, radical acceptance refers to fully and unconditionally accepting one's body without judgment, criticism, or the desire for it to be different. It involves embracing and making peace with one's body exactly as it is in the present moment.

Like body positivity and neutrality, this approach recognizes that bodies come in diverse shapes, sizes, and appearances and that there is no singular ideal or standard that everyone must adhere to. It involves letting go of societal expectations, comparing oneself to others, and striving for a specific body image. Instead, it emphasizes embracing the uniqueness and individuality of one's body.

Practicing radical acceptance in terms of body image means acknowledging and honoring the inherent worth and value of one's body, regardless of its perceived flaws or imperfections. It involves shifting the focus from external appearance to self-compassion, self-care, and overall well-being. Radical acceptance encourages individuals to cultivate a nurturing relationship with their bodies, treating them with kindness, respect, and gratitude.

## Activity 9.4 – Pick a Lens, Any Lens

Introducing group members to the various body image approaches allows them to consider which resonates most with them. These lenses can become part of their recovery skill sets and are useful in all situations where body image thoughts arise.

This activity teaches about the three aforementioned approaches and allows group members to practice applying them to their body image thoughts. Following that application, a discussion is generated to determine which felt most salient to them.

## Materials:

- Worksheet "Pick a Lens, Any Lens" (Appendix 9B)
- For in-person groups, provide paper and writing utensils for group members.
- For virtual groups, members can gather their writing materials or utilize electronic devices for the activity.

**Introduce** three body image approaches: body positivity, body neutrality, and radical acceptance. These approaches provide different perspectives on how individuals can relate to their bodies. Define each of them and give some examples of how to use them. Answer any questions about how they are similar and what makes them different.

Practice examining a distressing body image thought through three lenses: body positivity, body neutrality, and radical acceptance.

**Use** worksheet Appendix 9B to allow group members to practice using these approaches with their body image thought. Give members a few minutes to complete the handout individually. The last line of the worksheet asks them to select which approach resonated most with them.

**Reflect** as a group on how it felt to apply each of these approaches. Use the following discussion questions to generate discussion around their experiences.

- How would you describe the experience of considering one thought from different lenses or perspectives? What transformations or shifts did you observe as the original thought was explored through the lens of different approaches? How did these changes impact its power or significance for you?
- Did you notice any differences in the level of ease or difficulty when applying each approach? Can you elaborate on the factors that influenced your perception?
- Were there any particular approaches that evoked internal resistance or hesitation? If so, what do you think might have contributed to those feelings?

**Conclude** the discussion by inviting group members to reflect and share the approach that resonated with them the most. Validate that various approaches may land differently with each person, which is okay. These are recovery tools, and no one expects that every tool will be effective for everyone.

*Facilitators' Forum*

Paramount to the themes of body positivity, body neutrality, and radical acceptance is the idea that bodies are unique and that all body shapes, sizes, and abilities are valuable. How a person feels about that value begins to differentiate the approaches. In discussing body diversity, this conversation may circle back to themes centered around body and beauty standards, thoroughly addressed in Chapter 8. Facilitators will want to be familiar with these connections and able to bridge these topics skillfully should the conversation move in that direction.

## Physical Activity

The benefits of physical activity are indisputably plentiful; from stress reduction to improved sleep, disease prevention, and increased energy levels, there is no shortage of research confirming that even mild to moderate activity levels confer these benefits. However, as Connie Sobczak points out in her book *Embody*, there is a difference between being physically active for the benefits mentioned earlier and exercising with the intent to change the size or shape of one's body.[25] When the purpose of exercise becomes centered around unrealistic body ideals or when the compulsion to exercise is so strong that other forms of self-care are neglected, this potentially healthy practice can become detrimental to one's well-being. Exercise can also be a form of self-punishment in disguise, something that group members will sometimes not realize if this symptom has not been thoroughly addressed with their individual providers.

For a long time, it was considered best practice for physical activity to be reserved for fully weight-restored, if applicable, or fully recovered individuals. However, the professional stance on this has evolved, as Dr. Jennifer Gaudiani points out in *Sick Enough*.[26] Guiding individuals through the inclusion of physical activity during the recovery process is important and may actually improve retention in the process itself. Preventing movement until full weight restoration is achieved emphasizes the disordered belief that exercise's main function is to burn calories. When it is medically and psychologically safe, by permitting and supervising movement sooner in the recovery process, clinicians can help their clients gradually and skillfully incorporate movement back into their lives.[27] That being said, physical activity is a relevant topic to explore in the group as members may be in a proverbial gray zone concerning their relationship with exercise.

Reconnecting to the joy and spontaneity found through movement can be profound. Shifting away from militant exercise practices and toward a more intuitive, gentle approach to exercise allows for tuning into one's body and noticing what feels right, how hard to push, and when to stop. Abandoning numbers, steps, metrics, and other forms of tracking can be freeing for individuals who have felt stifled by rigid exercise routines and self-imposed rules.

Group facilitators should be mindful of those with compulsive exercise and exercise avoidance histories. This avoidant relationship is common among individuals who struggle with eating disorders and is often less talked about than the compulsive exerciser. The cause for this avoidance can be multifaceted. Perhaps there is a history of compulsive exercise followed by avoidance (the proverbial pendulum swinging in the other direction), discomfort or fear in moving one's body, or a long history of exercise not "working," particularly when performed for the purpose of weight loss.

In their acclaimed book *Intuitive Eating: A Revolutionary Anti-Diet Approach*, Evelyn Tribole and Elyse Resch provide pragmatic reminders for reclaiming joy through movement. Considering whether to include others in physical activity, such as taking a walk with a partner or friend, choosing something you really enjoy, or regularly varying the type of physical activity practiced, are ways to rediscover how to find pleasure through movement.[28]

### Activity 9.5 – Jumping for Joy and Bouncing for Bliss

Exploring one's relationship with physical activity can be impactful for individuals recovering from an eating disorder, regardless of their past experiences with excessive exercise, avoidance of exercise, or feeling disconnected from their bodies. It involves rediscovering or discovering for the first time exercise as a way to experience joy, have fun, and practice self-care.

This activity will prompt group members to consider whether their past exercise experiences have been positive or problematic. Where it is problematic, they will initiate the process of envisioning a new approach to exercise and identifying the necessary steps to cultivate this relationship.

### Materials:

- Worksheet "Jumping for Joy and Bouncing for Bliss" (Appendix 9C)
- For in-person groups, provide paper and writing utensils for group members.
- For virtual groups, members can gather their writing materials or utilize electronic devices for the activity.

**Initiate** discussion around how group members relate to physical activity with the following prompt:

> What is your relationship with exercise now? Has exercise played a role in your eating disorder?

**Use** the worksheet Appendix 9C, giving group members time to complete the prompting statements.

**Review** the worksheet as a group. Encourage group members to share their answers.

**Further** the discussion by asking:

- Were there any common answers, trends, or shared sentiments? What does this tell us?
- Can you identify any patterns or triggers leading to excessive exercise or avoidance?
- What steps are necessary to embark on a new relationship with exercise? How can you ensure it aligns with your recovery goals and promotes self-care?
- What strategies or techniques can you use to listen to and honor your body's needs and limitations during physical activity?
- What challenges or concerns do you anticipate as you explore a new relationship with exercise? How can you address or overcome them?
- How can the group support and encourage each other in reclaiming exercise as a positive and empowering aspect of recovery?
- How can you reimagine your relationship with exercise?

### Facilitators' Forum

It is important to recognize that a group member's decision not to engage in exercise, regardless of their recovery status, is a personal choice that deserves respect and validation. While physical activity can have numerous benefits for overall health and well-being, it is not the only path to recovery. Recovery from an eating disorder involves a complex interplay of various factors, including emotional, psychological, and behavioral aspects.

Some group members may have personal preferences, physical limitations, or different approaches to self-care that do not involve traditional exercise. It is crucial to create a space where individuals feel supported in their choices and are not pressured or judged based on their decision not to engage in exercise. Respecting and honoring each individual's autonomy and choices are fundamental in fostering a supportive and inclusive environment for everyone in the group.

## Notes

1  American Psychiatric Association. 2013. "Feeding and Eating Disorders." In *Diagnostic and Statistical Manual of Mental Disorders: DSM-5-TR*. Arlington, VA: American Psychiatric Association.
2  Pruzinsky, Thomas, and Thomas F. Cash. 2012. "Understanding Body Image: Historical and Contemporary Perspectives." In *Body Image a Handbook of Theory,*

*Research, and Clinical Practice*, edited by Thomas F. Cash and Thomas Pruzinsky. New York: Guilford Press.

3 Gaete, María Isabel, and Thomas Fuchs. 2016. "From Body Image to Emotional Bodily Experience in Eating Disorders." *Journal of Phenomenological Psychology* 47 (1): 17–40. https://doi.org/10.1163/15691624-12341303.

4 Rabinor, J. R., and Bilich, M. A. 2002. "Experiential Approaches to Changing Body Image." In *Body Image a Handbook of Theory, Research, and Clinical Practice*, edited by Thomas F. Cash and Thomas Pruzinsky, 469–477. New York, NY: Guilford Press.

5 Tiggemann, Marika, and Jessica E. Lynch. 2001. "Body Image across the Life Span in Adult Women: The Role of Self-Objectification." *Developmental Psychology* 37 (2): 243–253. https://doi.org/10.1037/0012-1649.37.2.243.

6 Atkinson, Melissa J., and Tracey D. Wade. 2019. "Mindfulness Training to Facilitate Positive Body Image and Embodiment Essay.". In *Handbook of Positive Body Image and Embodiment: Constructs, Protective Factors, and Interventions*, edited by Tracy L. Tylka and Niva Piran, 265–276. New York: Oxford University Press.

7 Segal, Zindel V., Williams, J., Mark, G., John D. Teasdale, and Jon Kabat-Zinn. 2018. *Mindfulness-based Cognitive Therapy for Depression: A New Approach to Preventing Relapse*. 2nd ed. New York: The Guilford Press.

8 Kelly, Allison C., Kathryn E. Miller, Kiruthiha Vimalakanthan, Jessica R. Dupasquier, and Sydney Waring. 2019. "Compassion-Based Interventions to Facilitate Positive Body Image and Embodiment Essay." In *Handbook of Positive Body Image and Embodiment: Constructs, Protective Factors, and Interventions*, edited by Tracy L. Tylka and Niva Piran, 265–276. New York: Oxford University Press.

9 Abbott, Bree D., and Bonnie L. Barber. 2010. "Embodied Image: Gender Differences in Functional and Aesthetic Body Image among Australian Adolescents." *Body Image* 7 (1): 22–31. https://doi.org/10.1016/j.bodyim.2009.10.004.

10 Alleva, Jessica M., Carolien Martijn, Anita Jansen, and Chantal Nederkoorn. 2013. "Body Language." *Psychology of Women Quarterly* 38 (2): 181–196. https://doi.org/10.1177/0361684313507897.

11 Webb, Jennifer B., Nichole L. Wood-Barcalow, and Tracy L. Tylka. 2015. "Assessing Positive Body Image: Contemporary Approaches and Future Directions." *Body Image* 14: 130–45. https://doi.org/10.1016/j.bodyim.2015.03.010.

12 Wood-Barcalow, Nichole L., Tracy L. Tylka, and Casey L. Augustus-Horvath. 2010. "'But I Like My Body': Positive Body Image Characteristics and a Holistic Model for Young-Adult Women." *Body Image* 7 (2): 106–116. https://doi.org/10.1016/j.bodyim.2010.01.001.

13 Frisén, Ann, and Kristina Holmqvist. 2010. "What Characterizes Early Adolescents with a Positive Body Image? A Qualitative Investigation of Swedish Girls and Boys." *Body Image* 7 (3): 205–212. https://doi.org/10.1016/j.bodyim.2010.04.001.

14 Avalos, Laura, Tracy L. Tylka, and Nichole Wood-Barcalow. 2005. "The Body Appreciation Scale: Development and Psychometric Evaluation." *Body Image* 2 (3): 285–297. https://doi.org/10.1016/j.bodyim.2005.06.002.

15 Wood-Barcalow et al., "But I Like My Body," 2010.

16 Fredrickson, Barbara L., and Tomi-Ann Roberts. 1997. "Objectification Theory: Toward Understanding Women's Lived Experiences and Mental Health Risks." *Psychology of Women Quarterly* 21 (2): 173–206. https://doi.org/10.1111/j.1471-6402.1997.tb00108.x.

17 Moradi, Bonnie, and Yu-Ping Huang. 2008. "Objectification Theory and Psychology of Women: A Decade of Advances and Future Directions." *Psychology of Women Quarterly* 32 (4): 377–398. https://doi.org/10.1111/j.1471-6402.2008.00452.x.

18  Prichard, Ivanka, and Marika Tiggemann. 2008. "Relations among Exercise Type, Self-Objectification, and Body Image in the Fitness Centre Environment: The Role of Reasons for Exercise." *Psychology of Sport and Exercise* 9 (6): 855–866. https://doi.org/10.1016/j.psychsport.2007.10.005.

19  Strelan, Peter, Sarah J. Mehaffey, and Marika Tiggemann. 2003. "Self-Objectification and Esteem in Young Women: The Mediating Role of Reasons for Exercise." *Sex Roles* 48: 89–95. https://doi.org/10.1023/a:1022300930307.

20  Prichard, I., and Tiggemann, M. 2008. "Relations among Exercise Type, Self-Objectification, and Body Image in the Fitness Centre environment: The Role of Reasons for Exercise." *Psychology of Sport and Exercise* 9: 855–866. https://doi.org/10.1016/j.psychsport.2007.10.005 Qualtrics. 2013. *Qualtrics Research Suite.* Provo, UT: Qualtrics.x

21  Tiggemann, Marika, Emily Coutts, and Levina Clark. 2014. "Belly Dance as an Embodying Activity?: A Test of the Embodiment Model of Positive Body Image." *Sex Roles* 71 (5–8): 197–207. https://doi.org/10.1007/s11199-014-0408-2.

22  Impett, Emily A., Jennifer J. Daubenmier, and Allegra L. Hirschman. 2006. "Minding the Body: Yoga, Embodiment, and Well-Being." *Sexuality Research and Social Policy* 3 (4): 39–48. https://doi.org/10.1525/srsp.2006.3.4.39.

23  Sole-Smith, Virginia. 2023. *Fat Talk: Parenting in the Age of Diet Culture.* New York: Henry Holt and Company.

24  Linehan, Marsha M., and Elizabeth T. Dexter-Mazza. 2008. *Clinical Handbook of Psychological Disorders: A Step-by-Step Treatment Manual.* 4th ed. (Edited by David H. Barlow), 379–420. New York: Guilford Publications.

25  Sobczak, Connie. 2014. *Embody: Learning to Love Your Unique Body (and Quiet that Critical Voice!).* Carlsbad: Gürze Books.

26  Gaudiani, Jennifer L. 2019. *Sick Enough: A Guide to the Medical Complications of Eating Disorders.* New York: Routledge.

27  Gaudiani, "Sick Enough," 2019.

28  Tribole, Evelyn, and Elyse Resch. 2020. *Intuitive Eating: A Revolutionary Anti-Diet Approach.* New York: St. Martin's Essentials.

# Appendix 9A – Exploring Body Functionality (for Activity 9.3)

Instructions:

Take some time to reflect on the following prompts and write down your thoughts and responses. Feel free to be as detailed and expressive as you would like. Once you have completed the worksheet, you can share your insights and reflections with the group if you feel comfortable doing so.

| Physical Capabilities | What are three physical capabilities or capacities of your body that you appreciate? Examples may include mobility and dexterity. | •<br>•<br>• |
|---|---|---|
| Biological Functions | Think about the biological functions of your body that contribute to your overall well-being. Examples may include the immune system or digestion. Write down three examples. | •<br>•<br>• |
| Senses | Reflect on your senses and how they enhance your experiences. Examples may include how smell can evoke memories, trigger emotions, and influence our perceptions of the world. Describe a moment when your senses allowed you to fully engage with the world around you. | |
| Creative Expression | How do you engage in creative expression beyond physical appearance? Write about an activity that allows you to express your creativity and connect with your body. Examples include singing or playing a musical instrument, dancing, yoga, painting, drawing, ceramics, acting, or writing poetry. | |

| Self-Care Practices | List two self-care practices you prioritize to support your overall well-being. Examples may include practicing mindfulness, joyful movement, and engaging in hobbies. | •  <br> • |
|---|---|---|
| Communication with Others | How do you use your body to communicate and connect with others? Examples may include a warm smile, a hug, or active listening by nodding, maintaining eye contact, and facing a speaker directly to show attentiveness and interest. Describe a situation where your body language or expressions played a significant role in conveying your emotions or connecting with someone. | |

# Appendix 9B – Pick a Lens, Any Lens (for Activity 9.4)

| Thought | ED Lens | Body Positive Lens | Body Neutral Lens | Radical Acceptance |
|---------|---------|--------------------|--------------------|--------------------|
| I have an ugly, round face. | My face is round because I'm so fat and I should lose weight. | Faces shouldn't all look the same and the roundness makes mine beautiful. | My face is unique and makes me look like me. My face is expressive and shows a full range of emotions. | My face looks round to me today and this is not good or bad. There is no "right" face shape. |
| | | | | |
| | | | | |
| | | | | |

Which approach resonates with you most? Why?

# Appendix 9C – Jumping for Joy and Bouncing for Bliss (for Activity 9.5)

Think of a form of exercise that you might engage in. Keeping this in mind, complete the following prompts:

- I know I would feel ready to do this because _____
- If I feel _____, this is a sign I should not do this activity right now.
- I might feel nervous or anxious about _____
- If I'm prioritizing my enjoyment, I would not _____ and would make sure to _____ while I do this.
- I will know this feels enjoyable if or when _____
- Something that would make this activity even more enjoyable would be
  _____
- I will know that I'm ready to stop this activity when _____
  _____
- When I think about doing this activity, I don't like that my eating disorder makes me think_____
- This biggest challenge or hurdle to implementing this activity in the way I've imagined here is: _____

# Chapter 10

# Fueling the Journey
## Healing the Relationship with Food Through Group Therapy

A common refrain in the world of eating disorder treatment is, *it's about the food, and not about the food*. Exploring values, barriers to change, and the connection with one's body is crucial in eating disorder recovery. However, addressing the complex relationship with food remains an essential aspect that cannot be overlooked. For some group members, clinging to specific food rules, rituals (which serve to reduce anxiety or discomfort around food), or labels (such as dairy-free or vegetarian) can be remnants of their eating disorder that last years past the initial treatment stage. Therefore, it becomes imperative to confront and navigate these lingering issues surrounding food to achieve lasting and sustainable recovery. By doing so, individuals can attain a healthier, more liberated relationship with food, fostering overall well-being and enhanced mental and physical health.

In addition to psychoeducation regarding normal eating, mindfulness, and the concepts of intuitive and mindful eating, this chapter incorporates experiential approaches, principles from Cognitive Behavioral Therapy, elements of Motivational Interviewing to elicit change talk, and Mindfulness-Based Practice to cultivate present-moment awareness. These evidence-based techniques and strategies help group members identify thought patterns that hinder their recovery and cultivate essential skills for lasting recovery.

### In a Relationship . . . With Food

As highlighted in Chapter 1, higher levels of care in eating disorder treatment primarily provide medical and nutritional stabilization for individuals struggling with eating disorders. The jarring changes in how one must eat in these treatment settings, whether a person needs to eat enough to support weight restoration or adjust to adequate, scheduled eating to circumvent bingeing, inform much of the conversation and work around food.

For someone returning to the outpatient setting from a higher level of care, that person starts to develop more of a relationship with food as more responsibilities are shifted back to them. This may encompass exploring

DOI: 10.4324/9781003430964-13

where or how they grocery shop, how much time to devote to food preparation, and what foods feel enjoyable and satiating. When subtle cues of pleasure return and bodily cues, such as hunger and fullness, are more apparent, it is easier to conceptualize how one thinks and feels about food. It follows that in an outpatient group, members are concurrently learning more about their relationship with food and challenging the lingering limitations their eating disorder imposes.

One benefit of the therapist and dietitian collaboration is that the outpatient group can be used to delve deeper into the participant's relationship with food. Certainly, the dietitian can probe further into the psychological underpinnings of someone's relationship with food and similarly, the therapist can further help that individual to explore their hunger and fullness cues. However, when these two professionals do this collaboratively and concurrently, it offers a more thorough and holistic experience for the group.

While celebrating personal victories with food, like adhering to meal plans during challenging weeks, holds significance and deserves acknowledgment, nutrition-focused groups also aim to provide a deeper understanding of how food can profoundly enrich our lives. Instead of eating to live, can one live to eat? Does a more peaceful relationship with food improve other aspects of life? Can one truly savor and enjoy food again while in recovery? The answer to these questions is a resounding *yes!*

Many factors influence the dynamic and ever-changing nature of our relationship with food as we navigate life's twists and turns. Various aspects such as income level, geographical location, marital status, and the different paths life takes can significantly impact what and how we eat. For instance, someone in eating disorder recovery transitioning from high school to college may experience newfound variety and access to diverse foods compared to their previous living arrangements at home. Similarly, a thirty-year-old woman who loses her job may need to scale back her food budget to conserve resources during challenging times. The group setting is a fitting place for individuals to share these changes and challenges and receive support from others.

For those in eating disorder recovery, it is vital to view this ever-changing food relationship landscape as a "given." Facilitators can empower group members to use their recovery skills to continue to make strides in recovery despite changing circumstances. Both clinicians, but particularly the dietitian, should be listening for these disclosures and ask how pertinent life changes have already or may in the future impact the individual's relationship with food.

## Activity 10.1 – Pick a Card, Any Card

It is normal for feelings toward specific foods and thoughts around them to change as eating disorder recovery progresses. What was once a fear food may now be perfectly acceptable food for someone, whereas other foods may continue to be challenging even years into recovery. This activity is meant to engage group members in a conversation about how our thoughts and feelings around food have evolved and elicit discussion about current attitudes toward food. This is a more food-specific activity, so it is an opportune time for the dietitian to step in to correct long-held inaccurate nutrition beliefs. Even though this activity starts out "turn based," the goal is for it to evolve into a broader group discussion in which everyone can participate.

## Materials:

- For in-person groups, the facilitators will need to prepare index cards with food names on them.
- For virtual groups, no materials are needed (see suggested modification).

**Place** several index cards (we recommend twice the number of group members, so for five members, put out ten cards) on a central table or surface. The cards should have one food written on them and be placed face down so that the food is not visible until the card is turned over. The listed foods should be a mix of traditional "safe" and "fear" foods; for example, pizza, broccoli, birthday cake, celery, Greek yogurt, chicken tenders, pumpkin pie, etc.

- For virtual groups, facilitators can try matching foods with a number (i.e., foods 1–10) and having group members select a number, which will then correlate with food that the facilitators will reveal. No physical card is needed.

**Invite** group members to take turns picking a card (or choosing a number) to reveal a food. They should read their food aloud to the group (or, if virtual, the food will be read by the facilitator).

**Ask** group members the following questions pertaining to the food on their card:

> What is your relationship with this food? Has it ever been a safe or fear food? Is it a food you enjoy? As you contemplate your recovery, what does your envisioned relationship with this food look like?

**Foster** discussion among group members, even if it is not their "turn," to cultivate relational learning. Use questions such as:

- When was the last time you had this food? Was it a memorable experience? Why or why not?
- Which emotions or feelings were elicited as the foods on the cards were revealed?

- Are there any positive experiences or breakthroughs you have had in your recovery that involve incorporating more or less of this food in your eating habits?
- Can you share any insights or personal growth you have experienced by reintroducing fear foods into your eating habits?

### Facilitators' Forum

Facilitators should use this activity with groups ready to speak to their *relationship* with foods rather than engaging in "food bashing" or propping certain foods up on a pedestal over other foods. If the conversation is veering toward demonizing or elevating foods over one another, the facilitators should remind group members that the goal of this activity is to reflect on the changing relationship with or attitudes toward a food over time. While this may entail sharing how a group member feels about the food, redirect them if they start categorizing foods as "good" or "bad."

## Activity 10.2 – Normal Eating Mission Statement

Clinicians often shy away from the word *normal* to honor the individuality inherent in all of us. With billions of people on the planet, it would be impossible to sum up one definitive norm for all eaters. Renowned Registered Dietitian and family therapist Ellyn Satter developed one of the best-known definitions of "normal" eating, which is easily accessible to share with your group if you so choose.[1] We have found her definition particularly helpful in our groups when members get stuck investigating the "right" way to eat.

In order to reflect on the recovery process, there is value in having group members consider what normal eating means to them and how aligned their habits are with the definition they create. This activity is intended to help the group arrive at the idea that it is challenging to pin down one norm for eating because people eat in such varied styles and ways. Especially when we consider cultural norms, religious customs, and varying accessibility to food, it is not surprising that different people will describe normal eating differently. Group facilitators should welcome and further this conversation. Encourage the group to discuss how an appropriate definition of normal eating encompasses more of an attitude toward food and nourishment than an assessment of right and wrong. The latter, also called dichotomous thinking, has been shown to correlate with eating disorders.[2]

## Materials:

- For in-person groups, a whiteboard (or similar) and writing utensil may be helpful in writing ideas down for the group to see.
- For virtual groups, screen sharing on any word processing program will allow the facilitators to take notes for the group to see.

**Prompt** the group by asking:

> You are tasked with coming up with a definition for normal eating. What belongs in this definition? What kind of message would you want to impart?

**Invite** group members to share their ideas and thoughts, which the group facilitators will write down (or type out) for group members to see.

**Facilitate** the formation of their ideas into one sentence, or a few if needed. Try to encompass as many ideas as the group comes up with in your definition. Then read the definition aloud.

**Reflect** on the definition the group has created by asking:

- When you think about your eating, are you a normal eater per the definition the group created? Why or why not?
- What aspects of the group's definition do you think you do well? Conversely, are there components of the group's definition that are still challenging for you to accept or put into practice?
- Is your definition of normal eating synonymous with being in eating disorder recovery? Why or why not?
- Does normal eating, according to our group's definition, feel attainable? What steps can you take to bring yourself closer to normal eating?

### Facilitators' Forum

Facilitators may further the discussion by probing into how the group's definition of normal eating contrasts with diet culture, addressed in Chapter 8. For example, they can consider whether their definition rejects the characteristics inherent in diet culture messaging. By asking how the group's definition diverges from diet culture influences, facilitators can continue to develop an understanding of how normal eating stands apart from diet culture.

## Finding Joy in Food Again

Eating is an inherently pleasurable behavior all humans must engage in to sustain life. Put simply, our brains receive chemical signals that this nourishment is good and necessary for life and thus, the positive feedback loop is perpetuated to continue prompting us to do this wonderful, essential thing: eat. Restrictive eating disorders derail this cycle and food becomes a threat, a source of anxiety or worry. Even bingeing may provide fleeting pleasure or relief, but distress will soon follow. True satisfaction is the last thing the eating disorder provides.

Connecting to a sense of pleasure and joy in food is not only a hallmark principle of the Intuitive Eating program as written by Evelyn Tribole and Elyse Resch in their book, *Intuitive Eating: A Revolutionary Anti-Diet Approach*, but also an aspiration for those in recovery.[3] Experiencing true food freedom, the ability to eat without a rigid plan, food rules, or compulsion, allows people to choose food based on what is available to them and what tastes or sounds good to them at that moment. They are the directors of their eating production.

### Discussion 10.1 – You're Invited to My Dinner Party

Many people have good memories of attending or hosting a party at some point in their life. Food is often involved in these celebrations. Asking group members to think about hosting a party where they are choosing the menu is a creative way to prompt them to think about food without interference from anxious thoughts such as, *Will I have to eat this?* Considering what would be fun to serve, to cook, or to present to their guests allows an opportunity to nurture a sense of enthusiasm around food that can precede joy.

This activity also introduces an element of mystery. Members may not immediately know where facilitators are going with this prompt until the connections start to be drawn for them. This intentional approach allows facilitators to better engage members who might mentally "check out" if they think they already know the activity's exact purpose or direction. It encourages participants to approach discussions and activities with an open mind, fostering a sense of curiosity and exploration. During our group sessions, we often received comments like, "I didn't know where you were going with this, but it was fun!" This highlights the positive impact of this approach.

**Invite** group members to consider the following prompt:

> Imagine that you are hosting a dinner party for a happy occasion. Try to imagine the occasion and who you would invite. Next, consider what food you would serve.
>
> What food would be fitting for the event? Would you serve something special to honor an attendee?
>
> Is there a dish you enjoy cooking or baking that you would be eager to serve?
>
> If you do not enjoy cooking, would you have a chef or favorite restaurant cater?
>
> Is there a certain dish that attendees would expect based on the occasion?

**Encourage** each member to share about their dinner party and what food(s) they would serve. After everyone has shared, further the discussion with questions such as:

- How did you feel considering this prompt? Was it a struggle to come up with your party menu? Was there any fear of liking the food too much?
- Was anyone reminded of good memories around those foods or of foods they like? If you remembered certain foods that used to be fear foods or binge foods, what emotions came up when you recalled being uncomfortable eating those foods? Is the same true now?
- How did you feel as you heard about the dinner parties that other group members contemplated? Did their ideas bring up any feelings for you? If so, which?

**Conclude** by providing context and explanation, if the group does not arrive at this themselves, by explaining that one of the goals for individuals in recovery is to replace the fear, shame, and guilt surrounding food with a sense of pleasure and contentment from food. Eating foods that they enjoy. Savoring flavors that please them. Questions to help the group come to this include:

- Did this activity help you connect with a sense of joy around food, whether from eating foods that you love or thinking about foods that put a smile on your face for one reason or another?
- Did this feel fun for you? How is that different from the way you usually think about food?

### Facilitators' Forum

While some group members may find their creative juices flowing during this activity because they are very socially or culinarily inclined, more socially apprehensive group members may struggle to engage with this prompt. In these cases, facilitators should be sensitive to their needs and offer alternative prompts that feel more approachable. For example, inviting one dear friend to a private dinner for a happy occasion or cooking a birthday dinner for a trusted friend or partner may feel more comfortable and appealing to those who feel uneasy in larger gatherings.

## Activity 10.3 – In the Eye of the Beholder

In Chapter 7, Activity 7.1 ("Shifting Perspective") utilizes ambiguous images to allow group members to practice seeing how one image can evoke a variety of interpretations. The same can be done with images of food. A person may view a food one way through the lens of their eating disorder, but when presented with an image of that food within a broader context, it can trigger an entirely different emotional reaction. This activity will allow group members to challenge their preconceived ideas about certain foods. In doing so, they will try to connect with the part of their mind that sees a more adaptable, and potentially more positive, relationship with them. By engaging in imaginative and interpretive exploration, group members pave the way for receptivity to food.

Additionally, this activity can serve as a convenient time-filler for brief intervals. Group facilitators have the flexibility to use only one image, taking just ten minutes of the group's time when necessary.

Similar to Activity 7.1, ambiguous food images can be found in print magazines, online, or even generated using artificial intelligence software. Some examples of food scenes include:

- A beach blanket spread out on the sand, adorned with an assortment of snacks including chips, cookies, and a bowl of fresh fruit
- A classic picnic basket opened to reveal an assortment of sandwiches, a container of pasta salad, and a selection of fruits
- An outdoor table at a street-side coffee shop adorned with a latte, a slice of cake, and a plate of pastries
- A kitchen scene with baking ingredients, including flour, eggs, chocolate chips, a stick of butter, and baking utensils

## Materials:

- For in-person groups, facilitators may distribute physical copies of an image or show it on a screen or tablet.
- For virtual groups, facilitators can show the image using screen share or a similar feature.

**Display** or distribute a food image. Ask the group to try to imagine a scene using the following prompt:

> Looking at this picture and using your imagination, put yourself in this scene. What do you see? What would you like to feel or experience? What would you like your attitude towards the food you see to be?

**Further** the discussion about their imagined food scenes by asking:

- Are any positive or negative memories or associations evoked as you look at these pictures?
- Is conceptualizing this food in this way different from how your eating disorder sees this food? If so, how?
- Does seeing this food in a different way, or telling yourself a new story about this food, open the door to thinking about this food differently? How could these insights help you develop a changed relationship with this food?

**Repeat** this with as many images as the facilitators would like.

**Conclude** the activity by reinforcing that reimagining a specific challenge with food, or telling oneself a different story about the context or situation, is a skill that group members can draw upon in challenging moments.

### Facilitators' Forum

Instead of using images for this activity, facilitators may use an imaginative scene for group members to ponder. For example, as an alternative to providing a picture of baking ingredients on the counter, the facilitators could say, "Picture yourself engaged in baking, mixing the ingredients and forming dough. How does it feel to create something from scratch? What emotions emerge as you engage with the process of baking?" In another example, instead of providing a picture of the coffee shop scene, the facilitators could say, "Visualize yourself at the coffee shop, taking a sip of the latte, enjoying the cake, or savoring a pastry. How does the atmosphere of the coffee shop influence your experience? What emotions arise as you try these foods?"

For this activity to run smoothly, group members must be able to imagine a different context to the image with the food aspect being a piece of the story, but not the entire story. They must be able to access other emotional cues and feelings that the images conjure, which may not be possible if they are too fixated on thoughts around the foods they see in the pictures. For this reason, this activity is suited for groups who are testing the waters of normalized eating and have experience eating a wide variety of foods in their recoveries.

## Intuitive Eating

The acclaimed book *Intuitive Eating: A Revolutionary Anti-Diet Approach* introduced the renowned non-diet approach in an accessible and palatable (no pun intended) way.[4] Even today, its updated editions continue teaching people how to connect with the joy and satisfaction of food while trusting their body's hunger, fullness, and pleasure cues. Being able to eat intuitively is often touted as the ultimate eating goal for someone in recovery, as eating disorder thoughts are diametrically opposed to this approach.

Individuals are often eager to begin the intuitive eating phase as it is a graduation, in a sense, from the structured meal plan. While some intuitive eating skills may be developed in a higher level of care, the outpatient setting is where one hones this ability. Therefore, outpatient groups are a fitting place to introduce the intuitive eating model or review it for those who have only been introduced to it in the past, whether in treatment or with their outpatient team.

One comment we often hear in groups is, "Intuitive eating sounds great, but I can't imagine ever being able to do this." In short, it feels unattainable. A nice thought, but impossible. Exploring this frustration in a group setting is an effective way to validate this common opinion and garner support from others in cultivating

Fueling the Journey 209

hope that it is possible. Facilitators must equip group members with the understanding that practicing intuitive eating comes later in eating disorder recovery for many and is simply harder for some than others. Knowing that struggling with intuitive eating does not mean anything is wrong with them can help relinquish the shame that some feel for struggling with developing this skill for so long.

Drawing on shared experiences in a group setting can be an effective way for members to see that intuitive eating is possible. When one person shares a "win" that they had in this area, it inspires others to believe that intuitive eating is achievable for them too.

### Discussion 10.2 – Wouldn't It Be Nice

Many individuals seeking eating disorder recovery aspire to become intuitive eaters. However, depending on their journey's unique and sometimes circuitous course, it can take considerable time to truly feel ready for and embrace intuitive eating. Even when someone feels prepared, transitioning from the security and comfort provided by a meal plan can often be challenging and unsettling. Using creative thinking and visualization allows cognitive flexibility to bridge the gap between how someone thinks now and how they would like their thinking to be. This discussion intends to help group members understand their barriers to eating intuitively by imagining what going through the motions would feel like.

This discussion uses two scripts to connect members with different aspects of being a tuned-in eater. The first touches on the sense of pleasure in eating and the second addresses identifying and listening to hunger and fullness cues.

**Read** the following scenario to the group. If they cannot imagine themselves in this situation quite yet, suggest that they imagine someone they know who has a good relationship with food (their dietitian, therapist, etc.).

> We are going to explore a scenario together. I want you to imagine that you are an intuitive eater. In this scenario, you are out to dinner with some co-workers. You like these people. You expect good conversation and one of your co-workers has been talking up this particular restaurant for weeks, but it's always booked. Luckily, someone was able to get a reservation. You open the menu. What happens next?

**Ask** group members to share how they would proceed in this situation. If prompting is needed or to further the group, consider asking:

- What factors do you consider as you make your order? What bodily signals or cues do you imagine you would feel?
- How is your order influenced by your comfort with intuitive eating and rejection of diet culture?

**Further** the conversation by asking group members to contrast this reflection with how they imagine this exercise would currently play out for them.

- How did imagining this situation feel different from any recent experiences you have had in restaurants?
- How would it feel to try this in real life? What is holding you back from trying?
- Are you willing to try practicing this? Why or why not?

### Scenario Two

**Read** the following scenario to the group. If they cannot imagine themselves in this situation quite yet, suggest that they imagine someone they know who has a good relationship with food (their dietitian, therapist, etc.).

> In our second scenario, I want you to imagine you are an intuitive eater again. It is an unseasonably pleasant spring day. You are at work, and it is your lunchtime. You feel your stomach rumble and you know you are hungry. You take your lunch outside instead of eating in your work break room or at your desk. You packed leftovers from last night's dinner, one of your favorite home-cooked dishes. You have some other sides with you to eat. You sit on a bench, open your lunch box, and begin eating. What happens next?

**Ask** group members to share how they would proceed in this situation. If prompting is needed or to further the group, consider asking:

- Assuming you packed plenty of food in your lunch, how would you decide when to stop eating?
- What bodily signals or cues do you imagine you would feel at the time of fullness?

**Further** the conversation by asking group members to contrast this reflection with how they imagine this exercise would currently play out for them.

- How do you currently decide how much to eat at a meal (i.e., avoidance of feeling full, judgment from the eating disorder, food rules around how much those around them eat, etc.)?
- Aside from bodily cues, is there other input influencing how much you might eat (i.e., next break, whether you can or cannot eat in your workspace, etc.)?
- What stops you from eating until fullness or stopping at fullness? Do we need to stop at fullness? What is holding you back from experimenting with this?

*Facilitators' Forum*

These discussion prompts require group members to imagine themselves as intuitive eaters, so be sure that intuitive eating has been adequately explained or that the group consists of individuals who are actively honing their intuitive eating skills. The dietitian should assess readiness for this discussion. If done with a group cohort prematurely, the discussion will fall flat as group members will struggle to move past envisioning themselves as intuitive eaters in the first place.

## Mindful Eating

The Center for Mindful Eating describes mindfulness as "the capacity to bring full attention and awareness to one's experience, in the moment, without judgment."[5] Mindful eating, therefore, is the application of mindfulness to the entire eating process. Just as Tribole and Resch's principles of intuitive eating promote a nonjudgmental and attuned relationship with food, so too does mindful eating involve a deliberate awareness and intentional choices that reflect one's inner wisdom instead of what diet culture may dictate.[6] However, the two are not synonymous approaches. Tribole and Resch write about this in their work. Intuitive eating is in fact a far more comprehensive attitude and approach, whereas mindful eating is used to depict an actual skill.[7]

Mindful eating is also an important skill to counter the strong influence of the eating disorder voice at eating times. A growing body of evidence shows that mindful eating may be a beneficial intervention for those struggling with eating disorders.[8] Being able to identify hunger is a necessary step in responding to it. Learning how to ground oneself by tuning into sensory stimuli and listening to one's body can help shift attention away from intrusive eating disorder thoughts and back to the present moment. A 2010 study found that deep breathing aided the recognition of hunger cues in a cohort of individuals with eating disorders across different diagnoses.[9]

Group facilitators should gauge where group members are along the continuum of mindful eating. If some group members follow a prescribed meal plan while others are still engaging in eating disorder behaviors, such as adhering to food rules, it may be worth delaying the introduction of mindful eating within the group. When eating disorder beliefs and thoughts are strong, there is a risk of mindful eating becoming ritualized or evolving into a new sort of food rule in itself, intensifying the restrictive nature of the eating disorder.

Consider someone sitting down to their lunch, picking up their apple and eating it slowly. They taste the flavors and listen to the feedback from their body, only to decide that their body feels full halfway through consuming the apple and they are not hungry for the remainder of their meal. In someone struggling with an eating disorder who may have disrupted hunger and fullness cues, it is clear that mindful eating could inadvertently reinforce food restriction. The dietitian can be an asset by picking up what group members share and evaluating readiness to delve into mindful eating within a group cohort.

Even with careful screening, it is important to acknowledge that group members may be in different stages of readiness when applying mindful eating practices. Facilitators will likely find that while some members come to the group with a more attuned eating style, others may struggle to connect with this inner wisdom. We have found that this mix of mindful eating abilities is beneficial; when someone with the ability to eat mindfully speaks about these experiences, it provides hope to those still cultivating this practice that it is possible *and* worth the hard work to get there.

When mindful eating is introduced or explored in a group, it is important to distinguish between a mindful eating exercise (such as Activity 10.4) and a more realistic application of mindful eating in everyday life. It is not possible, and arguably not beneficial for one's relationship with food, to be so thoroughly attuned to the complete sensory experience while eating. We might be enjoying a conversation with someone, catching up on some work, or scrolling through a screen as we eat. Facilitators should invite their group to have a rich conversation about mindful eating and how it can be pragmatically applied to modern life. For example, trying to tune in to sensory stimuli for the first few bites of food may be enough for someone to feel engaged in mindful eating. In contrast, others may enjoy a more deliberate pause at several points during an eating experience to consider sensory input and bodily cues.

Mindful eating does not have to be a rigid practice. Rather, it can be as gentle as just noticing eating disorder thoughts entering one's consciousness. Nonjudgmentally and intentionally, one can turn the focus back to what is happening in front of them and how their body feels.

### Activity 10.4 – Conscious Cuisine

Eating disorder thoughts may be intrusive and highly frustrating, but mindful eating is one skill that can aid the deflection of or sometimes escape from those thoughts. Shifting attention away from the eating disorder thought and toward one's experience in their own body is one way to build awareness of what is occurring outside of the eating disorder thought loop. This activity provides a simplistic prompt to practice mindful eating. It is a good place to start exploring this topic and is suitable for younger group members.

### Materials:

- Worksheet "Conscious Cuisine" (Appendix 10A)
- For in-person groups, provide writing utensils.
- For virtual groups, members can gather their writing materials or utilize electronic devices.

- For in-person groups, facilitators should provide a small portion of food to each group member. Common choices include a piece of chocolate or a slice of apple.
- For virtual groups, facilitators should ask group members to bring their small portion of food to the group. (It is beneficial to send an email prior to the group letting each group member know ahead of time so that everyone may participate.)

Each group member does not need to consume the same food for the activity. Having members choose different foods to foster more lively and descriptive conversation and processing may be more interesting.

**Read** the following script to the group. For clarity, we will use an apple as our food sample. Some modifications to the script may be necessary depending on the food you choose.

> We are going to engage in a sensory exploration of apples. It may be helpful to close your eyes as we do this activity. Pick up your apple slice. Feel it. Is it heavy or light? Smooth or bumpy? What else do you feel?
>
> Look at your apple. What colors do you see? Are there splotches or dots? Hues that blend or clash along the skin?
>
> Smell your apple. Do you smell any scent before taking a bite?
>
> Once you are ready, take a bite of your apple slice. Listen to the sound it makes as you take a bite, chew the skin and flesh of the apple, and swallow. Does the inside of the apple smell different than the outside? Does it look different than the outside?
>
> How would you describe the taste of your apple? Is it bitter, sweet, or tangy? Is the mouthfeel crispy or mealy? Is your apple juicy, and are your hands sticky?
>
> You may take as many bites of your apple slice as you would like.

**Direct** group members to Appendix 10A ("Conscious Cuisine") and ask that they write down some thoughts pertaining to their experience. Single adjectives are fine.

**Ask** group members to share observations or reflections, including intrusive thoughts or judgments that emerged during their experience.

**Further** the discussion with questions including:

- Were there any adjectives that surprised you or that you have not considered when you have eaten this food before?
- This exercise took a lot of deliberate thinking and self-attunement. You will not be able to apply this same level of attention to every meal you eat, nor is that necessarily the goal of being a mindful eater. Why then do we do exercises like this?
- How can you imagine yourself using this skill in your eating disorder recovery?

**Conclude** the activity by asking group members to share any other observations or insights pertaining to this exercise.

### Facilitators' Forum

The emergence of eating disorder thoughts as group members engage in this mindfulness exercise can make it challenging for some. The therapist should reinforce that it is okay to have anxious thoughts that may seem to interrupt the practice. The absence of those thoughts is not what makes one a mindful eater. The goal is not to get entangled in those thoughts and to allow one's awareness to return to the present moment.

## Food Rules and Rituals

Food rituals are compulsive food-related behaviors that a person uses, and anxiety ensues when those behaviors are not used. For instance, these could include cutting food into abnormally small pieces, counting each piece of food, or not letting foods on one's plate touch each other. Food rituals are not only seen in restrictive eating disorders; in fact, bingeing is sometimes ritualized. A person may have certain foods that they only binge on and for some, binges must follow an order, such as going from specific food to specific food.

Food rules are slightly different; these are arbitrary rules that dictate any aspect of how a person eats. Some food rules may apply to what a person eats, where food is purchased or obtained, or what nutritional criteria must be met to eat a certain food. Often these originate from messages gleaned from diet culture, but they could arise from what one was taught about food from parents, coaches, peers, or social media. Examples of food rules range from "I do not eat anything that contains over [number] of calories" to "I do not eat anything with [food ingredient]" to "I do not eat past [time]."

Some food behaviors may blur the line of a food rule or ritual. The underlying commonality is that a person would feel anxious and uncomfortable about breaking it. For this reason, this topic is especially suited for collaboratively led groups. While the dietitian can help challenge participants' beliefs that certain food rules are scientifically sound and necessary, the therapist should approach the discomfort and fear members will feel by breaking the rules or rituals.

Either food rules or food rituals are seen in virtually every eating disorder case. These hard and fast rigidities provide the structure and false sense of comfort that maintain the eating disorder. Sometimes a person will initially tell their providers that they do not have food rules or rituals, but with time and as they cultivate the ability to reflect on their eating disorder behaviors, these are typically unearthed rather quickly. In an outpatient group, members should already have insight into their use of food rules and food rituals and be willing to challenge them, if they have not yet begun to do so in their individual treatment.

## Activity 10.5 – Playing by My Own Rules

The eating disorder thrives within the construct of one's food rules or rituals, but taken out of context, they often make little sense and may even sound silly. Allowing group members to extract these from a meal setting and conceptualize them in a new way can provide an understanding that forms the foundation for challenging them with their actions.

## Materials:

- Worksheet "Playing by My Own Rules" (Appendix 10B)
- For in-person groups, provide writing utensils.
- For virtual groups, members can gather their writing materials or utilize electronic devices.

**Review** what makes a food rule or food ritual. Asking members to identify a few examples of each may be helpful to ensure proper understanding.

**Direct** group members to Appendix 10B and ask them to select one food rule or ritual that has been present in their eating disorder. Group members should take a few minutes to answer the questions.

- Appendix 10B provides a sample worksheet already filled out. Facilitators should note that the filled-in answers indicate common misinformation dispersed through our current diet culture.

Select one food rule or ritual employed by your eating disorder.
   Where did it come from? Why do you tell yourself you do this?
Is there a different reason you might really be doing this?
   What is in it for you not to use this ritual?
   What is stopping you from stopping?

**Encourage** group members to share their food rule or ritual and responses to the worksheet questions.

**Facilitate** discussion, encouraging group members to identify the diet myths in each other's rules and rituals. Use questions including:

- Did seeing your food rule or ritual on paper or saying it out loud help you gain perspective on how arbitrary or silly it is? If yes, could you use this as a tool when you have urges to use this rule or ritual?
- Were there any themes present in participants' answers to questions on the worksheet? If so, what might these commonalities indicate?

### Facilitators' Forum

The facilitators play a crucial role in helping group members make connections between their underlying beliefs and the rules and rituals they engage in. They should actively encourage and facilitate discussions in which group members challenge each other's continued adherence to these rules and rituals. Doing so promotes an environment of change and allows members to serve as supportive and healthy voices for one another. This collaborative approach fosters meaningful discussions and aids in the growth and transformation of each individual in the group.

## Notes

1 Satter, Ellyn. "What Is Normal Eating?" *Ellyn Satter Institute*, 2018. www.ellynsatterinstitute.org/wp-content/uploads/2017/11/What-is-normal-eating-Secure.pdf.
2 Lethbridge, Jessica, Hunna J. Watson, Sarah J. Egan, Helen Street, and Paula R. Nathan. 2011. "The Role of Perfectionism, Dichotomous Thinking, Shape and Weight Overvaluation, and Conditional Goal Setting in Eating Disorders." *Eating Behaviors* 12 (3): 200–206. https://doi.org/10.1016/j.eatbeh.2011.04.003.
3 Tribole, Evelyn, and Elyse Resch. 2020. *Intuitive Eating: A Revolutionary Anti-Diet Approach*. New York: St. Martin's Essentials.
4 Tribole and Resch. 2020.
5 "The Center for Mindful Eating." *The Center for Mindful Eating - Home*. www.thecenterformindfuleating.org/
6 Tribole and Resch, 2020.
7 Tribole and Resch, 2020.
8 Shaw, Ruth, and Tony Cassidy. 2021. "Self-Compassion, Mindful Eating, Eating Attitudes and Wellbeing among Emerging Adults." *The Journal of Psychology* 156 (1): 33–47. https://doi.org/10.1080/00223980.2021.1992334.
9 Hepworth, Natasha S. 2010. "A Mindful Eating Group as an Adjunct to Individual Treatment for Eating Disorders: A Pilot Study." *Eating Disorders* 19 (1): 6–16. https://doi.org/10.1080/10640266.2011.533601.

# Appendix 10A – Conscious Cuisine (for Activity 10.4)

| My food: | | | | |
|---|---|---|---|---|
| Touch | Taste | Smell | Sight | Sound |
| | | | | |
| Intrusive eating disorder thoughts or food judgments: | | | | |
| | | | | |

# Appendix 10B – Playing by My Own Rules (for Activity 10.5)

**Sample Worksheet**

| Food Ritual: Always eat fruit or vegetable component of meal first | | | | |
|---|---|---|---|---|
| **Where did this come from?** | **Why do I tell myself I do this?** | **Is there a different reason I might <u>really</u> be doing this?** | **What is in it for me not to use this ritual?** | **What is stopping me from stopping?** |
| I was told to always eat them first as a kid<br>Read online it was healthier to fill up on these foods first | To eat enough fruits and vegetables | To fill up on what I consider to be lower-calorie & healthier foods | Feel more present during meals<br>I can explore intuitive eating skills<br>I could eat what I enjoy most first | Afraid of eating too many calories if I start with other food groups first<br>Afraid I'll eat too much food that isn't healthy |
| **Food Rule: Don't eat past 7 PM** | | | | |
| **Where did this come from?** | **Why do I tell myself I do this?** | **Is my reasoning rooted in fact or feeling? If feelings, which?** | **What do I know is unreasonable or inaccurate about this rule?** | **What is stopping me from stopping?** |
| Read online that it's not healthy to eat late and I shouldn't eat after dinner | Feel disciplined<br>I don't want to feel heavy or full at night<br>It will affect my sleep | No – rooted in feelings of fear | Sometimes I feel hungry after 7 pm and preoccupied with thoughts of snacks<br>Sometimes can't sleep because I am hungry<br>I end up snacking anyway and feeling guilty | Worried about bingeing or eating too much at night<br>Worried about weight gain<br>Scared other people will judge me for snacking |

| Food Ritual: | | | | |
|---|---|---|---|---|
| Where did this come from? | Why do I tell myself I do this? | Is there a different reason I might <u>really</u> be doing this? | What is in it for me not to use this ritual? | What is stopping me from stopping? |
| | | | | |

| Food Rule: | | | | |
|---|---|---|---|---|
| Where did this come from? | Why do I tell myself I do this? | Is my reasoning rooted in fact or feeling? If feelings, which? | What do I know is unreasonable or inaccurate about this rule? | What is stopping me from stopping? |
| | | | | |

# Acknowledgments

Writing a book is an odyssey that is never taken alone, and we are profoundly grateful for the support and contributions of numerous individuals who have made this endeavor possible.

First and foremost, we would like to express our deepest gratitude to our dedicated peer reviewers, Erin Spotte, RD, LDN; Mindy Lais, Psy.D.; Sarah Ganginis, MS, RD, LDN; and Lisa D'Antonio, LCSW-C. Your commitment and generosity in taking the time out of your busy personal and professional lives to read and review our work was invaluable.

We extend our heartfelt appreciation to the network of supportive clinicians in our community who stood by us with unwavering encouragement to write this book. Your belief in the importance of this work motivated us to strive for excellence.

A special mention goes out to the talented individuals at T&F who played pivotal roles in bringing this book to fruition. To our dedicated editorial and Project Manager [Venkatesh Sundaram] at ApexCovantage, whose attention to detail and tireless efforts helped shape this book into its final form, we offer our sincere thanks.

We extend our heartfelt appreciation to our husbands, Richard and Hadar, for their patience, understanding, and support during the long hours and late nights dedicated to this project. Your love has truly been our anchor. We also want to extend our gratitude to our family members who shared in our excitement and believed in us as we embarked on this ambitious task.

Lastly, to the readers of this book, we hope that the knowledge and insights within these pages provide value and contribute positively to your understanding of eating disorder group therapy.

With gratitude,

Carolyn Karoll, LCSW-C, CEDS-S and Adina Silverman, MS, RD, LDN

# Index

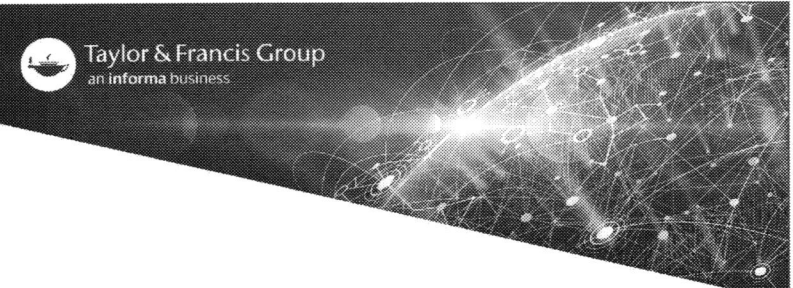
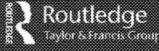
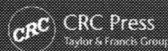

Printed in the United States
by Baker & Taylor Publisher Services